# CLINICAL GASTROENTEROLOGY

**Series Editor**

George Y. Wu
Division of Gastroenterology-Hepatology
University of Connecticut Health Center
Farmington, Connecticut, USA

More information about this series at http://www.springer.com/series/7672

Craig Rezac • Kristen Donohue
Editors

# The Internist's Guide
# to Minimally Invasive
# Gastrointestinal Surgery

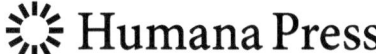 Humana Press

*Editors*
Craig Rezac
Virginia Hospital Center Physicians Group
Virginia Hospital Center
Arlington, VA
USA

Kristen Donohue
Robert Wood Johnson Medical School
Rutgers University
New Brunswick, NJ
USA

ISSN 2197-7399          ISSN 2197-7704 (electronic)
Clinical Gastroenterology
ISBN 978-3-319-96630-4          ISBN 978-3-319-96631-1 (eBook)
https://doi.org/10.1007/978-3-319-96631-1

Library of Congress Control Number: 2018963296

This Humana Press imprint is published by the registered company Springer Nature Switzerland AG
The registered company address is: Gewerbestrasse 11, 6330 Cham, Switzerland

*This text is dedicated to my wife Patrizia and my daughter Elena, my golf partners.*

# Contents

# List of Contributors

**Navid Ajabshir**  Department of Surgery, New Brunswick, Miami Beach, FL, USA

**Anthony Andreoni** Rutgers Robert Wood Johnson Medical School, New Brunswick, NJ, USA

**Kfir Ben-David** Department of Surgery, Mount Sinai Medical Center, Miami Beach, FL, USA

**Matthew T. Brady**  Department of Surgery, Division of Colon and Rectal Surgery, University of California Irvine Medical Center, Orange, CA, USA

**Igor Brichkov** Department of Surgery, Maimonides Medical Center, Albert Einstein College of Medicine, Brooklyn, NY, USA

**Michelle Y. Chen** School of Medicine, The George Washington University, Washington, DC, USA

**Shintaro Chiba**  Department of Surgery, Maimonides Medical Center, Brooklyn, NY, USA

**Jessica S. Crystal**  Department of Surgery, Rutgers Robert Wood Johnson Medical School, New Brunswick, NJ, USA

**Tomer Davidov**  Robert Wood Johnson Medical School, Rutgers University, New Brunswick, NJ, USA

**Anthony Delliturri** Department of Surgery, Maimonides Medical Center, Brooklyn, NY, USA

**Kristen Donohue** Robert Wood Johnson Medical School, Rutgers University, New Brunswick, NJ, USA

**Miral Sadaria Grandhi** Department of Surgery, Rutgers Robert Wood Johnson Medical School, New Brunswick, NJ, USA

Department of Surgery, Division of Surgical Oncology, Rutgers Cancer Institute of New Jersey, New Brunswick, NJ, USA

**Keith King** General Surgery, Rutgers Robert Wood Johnson Medical School, New Brunswick, NJ, USA

**T. Peter Kingham** Department of Hepatopancreatobiliary Surgery, Memorial Sloan Kettering Cancer Center, New York City, NY, USA

**Ioannis Konstantinidis** Department of Surgery, City of Hope Medical Center, Duarte, CA, USA

**Karl A. LeBlanc** Department of Surgery, Our Lady of the Lake Regional Medical Center, Baton Rouge, LA, USA

**Zinda Z. LeBlanc** Woman's Hospital of Baton Rouge, Baton Rouge, LA, USA

**Laleh Melstrom** Department of Surgery, City of Hope Medical Center, Duarte, CA, USA

**Raja R. Narayan** Department of Surgery, Stanford University, Stanford, CA, USA

Department of Hepatopancreatobiliary Surgery, Memorial Sloan Kettering Cancer Center, New York City, NY, USA

**Rachel E. NeMoyer** Rutgers Robert Wood Johnson Medical School, New Brunswick, NJ, USA

**Vincent Obias** School of Medicine and Health Sciences, George Washington University, Washington, DC, USA

**Alessio Pigazzi** Department of Surgery, Division of Colon and Rectal Surgery, University of California Irvine Medical Center, Orange, CA, USA

**Craig Rezac** Virginia Hospital Center Physicians Group, Virginia Hospital Center, Arlington, VA, USA

**Frank Senatore** Department of Medicine, Division of Gastroenterology and Hepatology, Rutgers-Robert Wood Johnson Medical School, New Brunswick, NJ, USA

**Haroon Shahid** Department of Medicine, Division of Gastroenterology and Hepatology, Rutgers-Robert Wood Johnson Medical School, New Brunswick, NJ, USA

**Daniela Treitl** Department of Surgery, Mount Sinai Medical Center, Miami Beach, FL, USA

**Gian-Paul Vidal** Robert Wood Johnson Medical School, Rutgers University, New Brunswick, NJ, USA

**Susannah Wise** Rutgers Robert Wood Johnson Medical School, New Brunswick, NJ, USA

# Chapter 1
# Introduction

**Kristen Donohue and Craig Rezac**

This text sets out to describe the many indications for and benefits of minimally invasive surgery (MIS) for the GI tract. This is by no means an exhaustive reference but meant to serve as an informative guide to appropriate patient selection and referrals. Minimally invasive surgery is often requested by patients, and we hope that this text serves as a reference for which patients would be candidates, what type of recovery and limitations to expect, as well as contraindications for minimally invasive approaches. We will briefly discuss the history and evolution of minimally invasive techniques. The general benefits of minimally invasive approaches will be referenced, and we will delve into more detail within individual chapters with regard to specific procedure types. Finally, there are many new and exciting tools on the horizon, and we will touch upon the future of minimally invasive GI surgery.

## A Brief History of Minimally Invasive Surgery

Minimally invasive surgery has come a long way from its origins. Hippocrates first mentioned a rectal speculum circa the year 400 BC; however, modern endoscopy was not used for patient care until the mid-1800s [1]. The first mention of entering full body cavities with a light source was by Jacobaeus in 1910. He coined the term "laparothorakoskopie" with examinations of both the thorax and abdomen [1]. Minimally invasive surgery as we see it today really began to take off in the 1980s, and there has been tremendous growth within the field in the last 30 years.

K. Donohue
Robert Wood Johnson Medical School, Rutgers University, New Brunswick, NJ, USA

C. Rezac (✉)
Virginia Hospital Center Physicians Group, Virginia Hospital Center, Arlington, VA, USA

© Springer Nature Switzerland AG 2019
C. Rezac, K. Donohue (eds.), *The Internist's Guide to Minimally Invasive Gastrointestinal Surgery*, Clinical Gastroenterology,
https://doi.org/10.1007/978-3-319-96631-1_1

The first laparoscopic appendectomy was performed by German gynecologist Dr. Kurt Semm in 1981 [2], and the first laparoscopic cholecystectomy was reported in 1987 by French surgeon Dr. Philippe Mouret [3]. This technique quickly spread from Europe to North America. In 1992 the US National Institutes of Health convened a Consensus Development Conference on Laparoscopic Cholecystectomy which estimated that about 80% of cholecystectomies were already being performed this way [4]. Today laparoscopy is used to treat innumerable intraabdominal pathologies of which appendicitis and gallstones are only the beginning.

Furthermore, robotic surgery is one of the more recent advancements in minimally invasive surgical technique. The first robot-assisted procedure was done in orthopedics in 1983 [5]. The use of robotics spread rapidly to urology and other pelvic procedures. The first FDA-approved use of robotics for general surgery was in 1993 by Yulin Wang [5]. Over time, different robotic platforms have been developed. Remote surgery is one additional potential benefit of robotics. Jacques Marescaux performed a robot-assisted cholecystectomy in 2001 on a patient in Strasbourg, France, 4000 km away from the surgeon in New York [5]. Today robotics is utilized by many different surgical subspecialties and has expanded from these initial uses to include thoracic and cardiac surgery and even ENT. This work will focus on GI surgery including hernias, gallbladder, liver, pancreas, and intestine.

## Potential Benefits of MIS

One of the greatest factors in growth for minimally invasive surgery has been patient interest and request. There are numerous benefits of minimally invasive surgery over open approaches. These include smaller incisions, less postoperative pain, less narcotic use, and less postoperative ileus. Additionally due to much of the above, patients experience faster return to daily activities including work [6].

## Relative and Absolute Contraindications

There are few absolute contraindications to minimally invasive GI surgery. Patients who cannot tolerate general anesthesia will not be able to undergo laparoscopic or robotic procedures. However, these are the exact patients that may benefit from advanced endoscopic interventions rather than large open surgical procedures if their disease process is amenable. Other contraindications include patients with multiple prior abdominal surgeries and significant scar tissue that prohibits sagely navigating the abdomen laparoscopically. Other potentially complicating factors include very large ventral hernias, inability to tolerate insufflation, and large liver obstructing the view of target anatomy.

Pregnancy, particularly first and third trimester, was traditionally viewed as relative contraindications to laparoscopy. However, the literature has more recently shown that laparoscopic surgery is safe during any trimester [7]. Both laparoscopic cholecystectomy and appendectomy have been done late in the third trimester without increased risk of preterm labor or death to the fetus [8].

## Future Directions

As minimally invasive surgery continues to grow, more advanced techniques and technology continue to arise. There are currently multiple "single-site" platforms for both laparoscopy and robotics. This eliminates the need for multiple small laparoscopic incisions, and allows the surgeon to operate through one slightly larger port, generally at the level of the umbilicus. The skin incision for these single-site surgeries is often not much larger than the traditional laparoscopic port site and is easy to hide within the umbilicus. The fascial incision is slightly larger than traditional laparoscopy or robotics, and this is associated with slightly increased incisional hernia risk compared to standard laparoscopic ports.

The future of minimally invasive surgery is looking to remove surgical scars and incisions in the skin all together. Natural orifice transluminal endoscopic surgery (NOTES) is a new technique where abdominal operations can be performed by passing an endoscope through a natural orifice (mouth, anus). The endoscope can then enter the abdominal cavity by making an internal incision through the stomach, vagina, colon, etc. to access the abdomen with no external incisions or scars [9].

## References

1. Radojcić B, Jokić R, Grebeldinger S, Meljnikov I, Radojić N. History of minimally invasive surgery. Med Pregl. 2009;62(11–12):597. https://doi.org/10.1179/acb.2010.032.
2. Semm K. Endoscopic appendectomy. Endoscopy. 1983;15:59–64.
3. Mouret P. From the first laparoscopic cholecystectomy to the frontiers of laparoscopic surgery: the future prospectives. Dig Surg. 1991;8:124–5.
4. Schlich T, Tang C. Patient choice and the history of minimally invasive surgery. Lancet. 2016;388(10052):1369–70. https://doi.org/10.1016/S0140-6736(16)31738-X.
5. Spinoglio G. Robotic surgery: current applications and new trends. Milano: Springer; 2015. https://doi.org/10.1007/978-88-470-5714-2.
6. Schwenk W, Haase O, Neudecker JJ, Müller JM. Short term benefits for laparoscopic colorectal resection. Cochrane Database Syst Rev. 2005;2:CD003145. https://doi.org/10.1002/14651858. CD003145.pub2.
7. Weiner E, Mizrachi Y, Keidar R, Kerner R, Golan A, Sagiv R. Laparoscopic surgery performed in advanced pregnancy compared to early pregnancy. Arch Gynecol Obstet. 2015;292:1063–8.
8. Affleck DG, Handrahan DL, Egger MJ, Price RR. The laparoscopic management of appendicitis and cholelithiasis during pregnancy. Am J Surg. 1999;178:523–9.
9. Baron TH. Natural orifice transluminal endoscopic surgery. Br J Surg. 2007;94(1):1–2. https://doi.org/10.1002/bjs.5681. PMID 17205508.

# Chapter 2
# Endoscopic Interventions

**Frank Senatore and Haroon Shahid**

## Introduction

Endoscopy is a procedure that allows the examiner to look inside a hollow organ or cavity in the body. It consists of a flexible tube with a light delivery system utilizing a lens to transmit an image to a camera. Gastroenterologists employ the use of many different types of endoscopes to aid in the diagnosis and management of many unique conditions of the digestive tract. The endoscope is maneuvered through the gastrointestinal tract under direct visualization on a projected monitor. They contain an air delivery system to insufflate the gastrointestinal tract lumens, as well as several channels for water and insertion of tools and devices used during endoscopy.

While a specific date is difficult to identify for the beginning of modern endoscopy, Philipp Bozzini is credited for achieving the first attempt to visualize the interior body and by most is considered the father of endoscopy. The first endoscope was made in Mainz, Germany, in 1806, and Antonin Jean Desormeaux is recognized for performing the first successful operative procedure using an endoscope.

Initially shunned, the endoscope grew in prominence following the advent of electricity, with its first commercial use coming in 1865 in Dublin, Ireland, by Francis Cruise. Three years later, Adolph Kussmaul became the first person to perform endoscopy in the stomach of a human. As the locations for the use of an endoscope increased, designs for specialized endoscopes tailored to different parts of the

F. Senatore (✉) . H. Shahid
Department of Medicine, Division of Gastroenterology and Hepatology, Rutgers-Robert Wood Johnson Medical School, New Brunswick, NJ, USA

© Springer Nature Switzerland AG 2019      5
C. Rezac, K. Donohue (eds.), *The Internist's Guide to Minimally Invasive Gastrointestinal Surgery*, Clinical Gastroenterology,
https://doi.org/10.1007/978-3-319-96631-1_2

body were envisioned. In 1881, Johann von Mikulicz created the first gastroscope which was used to visualize the esophagus, stomach, and small intestine.

The twentieth century saw the focus shift to improving the quality and resourcefulness of endoscopes. In 1932, the first flexible endoscope was developed. In 1957, the first fiberoptic endoscope was built, and the ability to steer the end of the endoscope came shortly thereafter. The 1960s saw the advent of automatic air insufflation, paving the way for new therapeutic devices to be invented, including thermal coagulation devices. By the 1970s, millions of procedures were being performed with endoscopes in the USA alone.

As endoscopes continued to be refined, videoscopes which were electronic endoscopes with a built-in video camera allowing for conversion of an image to an electric signal that could be displayed on a TV monitor were introduced. Ultrasonic endoscopes followed, with a transducer at their tip to allow deeper levels of tissue to be evaluated. Finally, in 2002, high-definition systems were devised to improve image quality and assist in more accurate diagnosis. Today, there are dozens of different endoscopes used in gastroenterology alone to aid in the diagnosis and management of digestive diseases.

Some of the most common indications for endoscopy include symptoms such as abdominal pain, nausea, vomiting, difficulty swallowing, weight loss, and gastrointestinal bleeding. Endoscopy is also indicated for many common diagnoses including anemia, cancers of the digestive tract, malabsorption, and infections. Finally, there are many common therapeutic interventions for which endoscopy is indicated including removal of foreign bodies, control of bleeding, diagnosing and managing neoplasms, and feeding tube placement.

Overall, gastrointestinal endoscopy is a minimally invasive procedure associated with reduced risks when compared to surgery, allowing for safe implementation in most patient populations. The indications for endoscopy and possible diagnostic and management modalities continue to grow within the field. Herein, we will discuss multiple conditions and locations within the digestive tract in which different forms of endoscopy and endoscopic techniques are routinely performed.

## GI Bleeding

### Peptic Ulcer Disease

Bleeding from peptic ulcer disease is a common explanation for patient's presenting with hematemesis, melena, and anemia. While the majority of patients with peptic ulcers will stop bleeding spontaneously, a cohort of patients will require endoscopic therapy. During upper gastrointestinal endoscopy evaluation, ulcers are classified based on their gross appearance to determine the need to endoscopic therapy. This classification, known as the Forrest classification, includes ulcers with spurting or oozing hemorrhage, nonbleeding visible vessels, and adherent clots. These peptic ulcers all require endoscopic therapy, whereas ulcers with a flat pigmented spot or clean base do not require endoscopic therapy.

There are several types of endoscopic therapies for peptic ulcer disease. Consensus guidelines recommend dual therapy during endoscopic treatment, which always includes the injection of epinephrine. A small injection needle is inserted through the endoscope channel with an epinephrine-filled syringe on the opposite side. Then, the needle is inserted into the ulcer site, and a 1:10,000 solution of epinephrine is administered. Epinephrine injection is relatively simple to deliver and often makes the bleeding ulcer site cleaner for the subsequent application of additional therapies. Epinephrine causes vasoconstriction of the bleeding vessel and allows for mechanical compression. Epinephrine injection is a safe modality but does carry a risk of tachycardia and arrhythmias.

Following this, thermal therapy or hemoclips are applied to the ulcer site. For peptic ulcer disease bleeding, thermal therapy is used in the form of a bipolar cautery probe. This probe is inserted through the endoscope channel and applies a high-frequency electrical current to the peptic ulcer to coagulate the surrounding tissue. The probe is applied with direct contact on the peptic ulcer, and firm pressure is applied for approximately 10 s, while the current is delivered. Based on the size of the ulcer and the amount of bleeding, this therapy can be applied several times. The main risk associated with this treatment modality is perforation, although this is quite rare [1, 2].

Hemoclips, also called endoclips or hemostatic clips, are steel clips that are inserted through the endoscope channel with a control device on the opposite end to open, close, and release the clip. Tissue around the peptic ulcer is grasped on either side of the bleeding site, and the hemoclip is closed, compressing off the surrounding area of bleeding. The endoclip tightly opposes the tissue, and then it is released from the endoscope. Unlike thermal therapy, hemoclips do not damage the ulcer tissue. More than one hemoclip may need to be placed based on the size of the ulcer and degree of bleeding. Hemoclips may also serve a dual purpose in being a radiopaque marker, should endoscopic intervention be unsuccessful and surgical or angiographic treatment be necessary.

## Angioectasias

Angioectasias, also known as arteriovenous malformations (AVM), angiodysplasias, and vascular ectasias, are aberrant blood vessels that have a fern or spider veinlike appearance within the gastrointestinal tract. They are the most common vascular condition found in the gastrointestinal tract, associated with advanced age and several genetic disorders. Angioectasias are also associated with several common medical conditions including end-stage renal disease, aortic stenosis (called Heyde's syndrome), and von Willebrand disease. Angioectasias can occur anywhere in the GI tract but tend to more commonly occur in the small intestine. Bleeding from angioectasias typically presents in the form of anemia or occult gastrointestinal bleeding.

Argon plasma coagulation (APC) is the most commonly used endoscopic modality to treat bleeding angioectasias. This technique employs an electrical current in a slightly different approach. A probe is inserted through the endoscope channel and directed at the angioectasia but kept at a short distance from the lesion.

Argon plasma is released from the probe and ionized by high-voltage discharge, resulting in an electrical current conducted through the argon plasma gas. This coagulates the lesion and surrounding tissue. It is generally considered to be a more superficial treatment approach than bipolar cautery, reducing the risk of perforation. Frequently, even if angioectasias are encountered without active hemorrhage, they are still treated as they can bleed in the future [3].

## Variceal Bleeding

Varices are dilated submucosal veins that result from portal hypertension. They are commonly found in patients with cirrhosis and most commonly occur in the esophagus and stomach. Variceal hemorrhage is a severe and life-threatening form of gastrointestinal bleeding. Patients typically present with large volume hematemesis, melena, and sometimes hematochezia due to rapid transit bleeding. Frequently these patients are hemodynamically unstable and require emergent endoscopic intervention.

Endoscopic band ligation is the hallmark of treating esophageal varices. It involves placing small elastic bands around varices. The band ligator is placed around the end of the endoscope and advanced to the location of the esophageal varices. These dilated veins are suctioned into the band ligator device, and elastic bands are fired one at a time, effectively wrapping around the base of the esophageal varix. Once secured, the band ligates the tissue and causes necrosis. Eventually, the band and necrotic tissue fall off when the underlying tissue fibroses. This approach is not only used for patients with active variceal hemorrhage but is also used prophylactically in patients with large esophageal varices [4].

In patients with variceal bleeding refractory to endoscopic band ligation, balloon tamponade placement can be used. The Sengstaken–Blakemore tube and Minnesota tube are the most common balloon tamponade tubes. They have a deflated esophageal and gastric balloon. The tube is advanced into the stomach; the gastric balloon is inflated with air and pulled up to the gastroesophageal junction. The outer portion of the tube is fastened to a device to maintain traction. The esophageal balloon can also be inflated if the bleeding persists. This is intended to be used as a temporizing measure to control variceal bleeding, until more permanent interventions can be initiated.

Sclerotherapy is an alternative for the treatment of variceal bleeding that consists of the injection of a sclerosant solution into varices, causing the destruction of tissue. It is delivered using an injection needle that is inserted through the endoscope channel. Ethanolamine and sodium tetradecyl sulfate are two commonly used sclerosants.

Gastric varices are more difficult to control endoscopically. Cyanoacrylate glue injection has proven to be effective in treating gastric varices although rebleeding can occur in over 20% of patients. More recently, endoscopic ultrasound has been utilized to deploy stainless steel coils into the gastric varices for varix obliteration with complete obliteration of fundal varices in up to 93% of cases [5].

## Hemorrhoidal Bleeding

Hemorrhoidal bleeding is one of the most common causes of lower gastrointestinal bleeding, commonly occurring in patients with constipation. While often self-limiting, hemorrhoids can progressively worsen causing debilitating symptoms of pain, pruritus, and, in chronic cases, anemia. In circumstances where conservative approaches such as topical treatment are ineffective, minimally invasive treatment options are available.

Rubber band ligation is a simple outpatient treatment option for patients with internal hemorrhoids. It is the most common procedure used to treat hemorrhoids, utilizing a rubber band that is applied to the base of a hemorrhoid to interrupt its blood supply, causing it to become ischemic and then necrotic before falling off. The rubber band is delivered via an anoscope, and currently there are several devices available to apply the rubber band. These include traditional forceps and suction ligators, which use different types of suction to obtain larger amounts of hemorrhoidal tissue within a drum, over which the rubber band is fired. It is indicated for patients with grade two or three internal hemorrhoids. The entire process normally takes less than 1 month from the procedure to the removal and healing of the hemorrhoid. Overall, rubber band ligation is considered to be one of the safest and most effective forms of hemorrhoidal treatment.

Sclerotherapy is an alternative to hemorrhoid treatment as well. It is indicated for patients with grade one to three internal hemorrhoids; however, it is associated with higher rates of recurrence than rubber band ligation. Two conditions in which sclerotherapy is indicated over rubber band ligation are in patients with elevated bleeding risks and who are immunocompromised.

Newer technology to treat hemorrhoids includes the implementation of infrared coagulation, monopolar cautery, bipolar diathermy, laser photocoagulation, or cryosurgery. These techniques all employ the principle of causing coagulation and necrosis within the hemorrhoids, leading to fibrosis. They are indicated for patients with grade one to two internal hemorrhoids.

The HET Bipolar System is a new modified anoscope used in the treatment of internal hemorrhoids associated with bleeding and prolapse. This system allows for internal hemorrhoids to be positioned within the device and treated with bipolar energy to ligate hemorrhoidal feeding vessels [6].

## Diverticular Bleeding

A diverticulum is a saclike protrusion of the colonic wall, normally formed from a weakening in the colon wall in conjunction with increased colonic pressure. It is age related but can be more prevalent in patients with constipation. A complication of diverticulosis is diverticular bleeding, which normally presents with painless hematochezia. The bleeding is brisk, large volume and normally transient, as it is arterial bleeding within a diverticulum. Diverticular bleeding is almost always self-limiting, although rarely endoscopic therapy is necessary to control bleeding.

Both hemoclips and thermal therapy in the form of bipolar cautery can be used to treat an actively bleeding diverticulum. Hemoclips can be applied in one of two ways to treat diverticular bleeding. They are directed at the bleeding vessel within the diverticulum to compress the active site of hemorrhage or across the mouth of the diverticulum to pinch it closed. Bipolar cautery targets the bleeding vessel within the diverticulum but coagulates the vessel and surrounding tissue to halt the bleeding. Hemoclips are often considered a safer option than thermal therapy for treating active diverticular bleeding, as these diverticula are thin-walled, and associated with higher rates of perforation than normal colonic tissue [7]. It is also worth mentioning that diverticula can form throughout the small intestine as well. If bleeding occurs, similar therapeutic approaches can be instituted.

## *Enteroscopy*

While esophagogastroduodenoscopy and colonoscopy allow for the visualization and aforementioned treatment implementation approaches, many pathologic disorders including bleeding can occur within the small intestines. To access the small bowel, several endoscopes are employed.

Small bowel enteroscopy involves the use a slightly longer and wider endoscope (compared to esophagogastroduodenoscopy). While esophagogastroduodenoscopy can access up to the second portion of the duodenum, small bowel enteroscopy can access the third and fourth portion of the duodenum, as well as the proximal and mid jejunum. This enteroscope contains the same channels to accommodate the treatment devices used in gastrointestinal bleeding.

Single-balloon enteroscopy involves the use of an enteroscope with an overtube on the distal end containing a silicon balloon. This balloon can be inflated and deflated to aid with enteroscope advancement through the small bowel. Typically, this enteroscope allows for access through the distal jejunum and into the proximal ileum. Double-balloon enteroscopy is similar to single balloon but employs two silicon balloons with one attached to the overtube and the other attached to the endoscope. This allows for access to the entire small bowel to the terminal ileum. Spiral enteroscopy uses an overtube that acts as a screw, which pleats the small bowel over the endoscope and can reach similar depths as a double-balloon enteroscopy but in a shorter duration [8].

When enteroscopes are used, the most distal site that is reached is normally marked with a tattoo for future reference. An injection needle is inserted through the enteroscope, and India ink is injected into the mucosa, staining it blue. This permanent tattoo can also be used for marking areas throughout the upper and lower gastrointestinal tract.

## Tissue Sampling

When performing endoscopy, whether it be esophagogastroduodenoscopy, enteroscopy, or colonoscopy, abnormalities are frequently encountered that require histological examination to confirm the diagnosis. These abnormalities range from erythema of mucosa to polyps to malignant-appearing masses. Tissue sampling in the form of biopsy is the most commonly used interventional modality in endoscopy to allow for a tissue specimen to be examined histologically. These samples can not only be sent for histological examination but also for cytologic and microbiologic analysis.

Biopsy consists of a steel forceps with two claws opposing each other that close to a tight seal. It is placed through the endoscope channel, advanced to the target tissue, opened, and closed. The biopsy forceps is then pulled back from the tissue, acquiring the tissue in a pinch biopsy approach. This technique is used to sample mucosal lesions and is normally not effective for submucosal or deeper lesions. Once the specimen is obtained, the biopsy forceps are withdrawn from the endoscope channel, and the tissue is placed into a specimen container for analysis.

Brushing is another form of tissue acquisition that is commonly used to identify mucosal plaques concerning for infection or masses concerning for malignancy. A brush inside a sheath is inserted in the endoscope channel and advanced to the target tissue. The head of the brush is then moved outside of the sheath, and the tissue is gently brushed collecting cells and specimen. The head of the brush can then be withdrawn into the sheath, and the entire device removed for the specimen to be placed in a collection container.

Polypectomy is a maneuver in which polyps are removed from the mucosal lining of the gastrointestinal tract. The method by which polys are removed depends primarily on the size of the polyp. Biopsy forceps are commonly used for polyps less than 4 mm, as the entire polyp can be successfully resected in one maneuver. Larger biopsy forceps including jumbo forceps are also used in a similar manner and can remove polyps less than 6 mm in size.

Snare polypectomy is a technique used to resect larger polyps. It involves a metal snare inside a sheath that is inserted through the endoscope channel to the tissue of interest. The opposite end of the snare has a control to allow for opening and closing. The snare is opened around the polyp and then slowly closed until the entire polyp is captured within it. The polyp is then cut either by the snare itself, called cold snare, or cut with electrocautery, called hot snare, to resect the tissue. In general, polyps less than 1 cm are removed with cold snare, and polyps greater than 1 cm are removed with hot snare [9].

Endoscopic mucosal resection (EMR) is a technique used for large and/or flat polyps that separates the mucosal layer from the muscularis propria. An injection needle is inserted through the endoscope channel, and saline solution is injected into the mucosal layer, lifting the polyp as a fluid cushion is created beneath it. Normally 1–4 ml or fluid is used. Sometimes other solutions are used including dextrose, glycerol, fructose, sodium hyaluronate, and hydroxypropyl methylcellulose. Recently new products have been created that include methylene blue in the solution to stain the submucosa and therefore better differentiate the tissue layers. Once the tissue is lifted, a hot snare is used to remove the polyp. On occasion, the polyp will be so large or irregular that all of it will not be able to be removed with a single hot snare. In that case, the hot snare is used additional times to remove the remaining polyp tissue, a process called piecemeal polypectomy.

Endoscopic submucosal dissection (ESD) is an advanced technique that uses a needle-knife inserted into the endoscope channel to dissect through the submucosal layer of tissue around a mass in the gastrointestinal tract. It is indicated for the removal of mucosal or submucosal masses irrespective of size and has the benefit of being used as a minimally invasive approach to early gastrointestinal cancers. ESD does carry a higher risk of bleeding and perforation but affords the ability to get an en bloc resection of a large polyp or early cancer. It is estimated that the recurrence rate after piecemeal EMR of a large polyp is about 20–30% vs about 1% with ESD. ESD usually is only offered by highly skilled endoscopists at tertiary care referral centers [10].

## *Endoscopic Ultrasound with Fine Needle Aspiration (FNA)*

Endoscopic ultrasound is a specialized endoscopic procedure involving an endoscope with an ultrasound probe, called an echoendoscope. The echoendoscope is advanced to many areas within the gastrointestinal tract allowing for ultrasound to be performed directly beside organs and masses that are adjacent to the luminal GI tract. This minimally invasive technique provides detailed and extremely accurate imaging to aid in the diagnosis and management of many conditions. Some of the indications for endoscopic ultrasound include staging of masses and diagnosing of biliary abnormalities.

Endoscopic ultrasound has the unique capability of being able to guide a biopsy needle into lesions for sampling. Many of these lesions are too small to be characterized or are located in regions that prevent percutaneous biopsy. A device with a biopsy needle is inserted through the echoendoscope channel and aligned with the end of the ultrasound probe. The biopsy needle tip is located via ultrasound and inserted into tissue for sampling under direct, constant visualization with ultrasound. The ultrasound provides the added benefit of assuring the correct structure is sampled and vascular structures are avoided using Doppler imaging. A fine needle aspiration (FNA) or fine needle biopsy (FNB) can be performed. Indications for endoscopic ultrasound with FNA/FNB include sampling of mucosal or submucosal lesions, sampling of peri-intestinal structures like masses and lymph nodes, fluid aspiration, and organ sampling (including liver biopsy). Overall, complication rates from this procedure are very low, and it is very well tolerated.

## Obstructing Lesions

### *Dilation*

Dilation is an approach used to treat strictures within the gastrointestinal tract. The most common location of gastrointestinal strictures is within the esophagus, causing patients to present with symptoms of dysphagia. Esophageal strictures are frequently associated with gastroesophageal reflux disease, eosinophilic esophagitis, caustic ingestions, prior radiation exposure, or malignancy.

Dilation can be accomplished in the form of mechanical or balloon dilators. Mechanical dilators are normally passed blindly or over a guidewire that is initially inserted endoscopically passed the narrowed region. One by one, plastic dilators each progressively larger in diameter are passed over the guidewire, subsequently moving through the narrowed region. Each dilation enlarges the lumen diameter slightly, until the narrowed region is widely patent. Balloon dilators are normally inserted through the endoscope channel and advanced past the strictured region. They are then inflated with pressurized water to a progressively larger diameter until the area is widely patent. Depending on how narrowed the region is, repeat dilations may be required at subsequent sessions, as the risk of perforation increases as the diameter to which a stricture is dilated increases. Dilation does not always permanently treat strictures, and over time, even benign strictures frequently recur, requiring repeat treatment.

## Stenting

Masses may be encountered in the gastrointestinal tract lumen that are large and obstructing. When found in the esophagus, small intestine, and colon, stenting may be used to temporarily relieve the obstruction before more definitive treatment or for palliative purposes. The most commonly used stents for the gastrointestinal lumen are self-expandable metal stents, but plastic and biodegradable stents exist.

Metal stents come in varieties of uncovered, partially covered, or fully covered stents. Covered stents tend to resist tumor ingrowth and have the potential to be removed but migrate more frequently. Uncovered stents are much less likely to migrate, but tumors can grow within them eventually causing repeat obstruction. Plastic stents are newer stents that have been developed for benign diseases in the gastrointestinal tract, and biodegradable stents are currently in research for benign conditions or as part of neoadjuvant therapy prior to definitive surgery.

A catheter and guidewire are passed through the obstructing region done under either endoscopic or fluoroscopic guidance. The catheter is then removed, and the stent is passed over the guidewire. The stent is then deployed and the guidewire is removed. Once the stent is deployed, it slowly expands against the obstructing tissue, which anchors the stent in place. This expansion can take several days to become complete. Complications associated with stenting include perforation, bleeding, stent migration, and stent obstruction [11].

## Esophagus

### Gastroesophageal Reflux Disease (GERD)

GERD is a condition that develops when contents in the stomach are refluxed into the esophagus, causing common symptoms of heartburn and regurgitation [12].

Endoscopic therapies in GERD have both diagnostic and therapeutic advantages. To confirm the diagnosis of GERD in patients with equivocal symptoms or response to initial treatment, a Bravo pH monitor can be used. To perform this study, an esophagogastroduodenoscopy is performed, and the junction of the esophagus and stomach is identified. The Bravo pH monitor is attached to the esophageal mucosa approximately 6 cm above the gastroesophageal junction. This device monitors the amount of acidity in the esophagus and communicates with an external device recorder over 24–48 h. The Bravo pH monitor falls off after several days and passes through the gastrointestinal tract.

Transoral incisionless fundoplication (TIF) is a minimally invasive treatment for GERD using the EsophyX (EndoGastric Solutions, Redmond, WA, USA) device. It is performed inside the stomach and creates a valve by folding the fundus of the stomach up and around the distal esophagus. This fundoplication is held in place by multiple fasteners that are implanted into the esophageal and stomach tissue. This minimally invasive procedure can also simultaneously reduce small hiatal hernias (less than 3 cm in size). The overall effect is limiting the reflux of stomach contents into the esophagus. Over a 3-year follow-up period, 90% of patients had elimination of regurgitation, and 71% of patients had discontinued PPI therapy [13].

## Barrett's Esophagus

Barrett's esophagus is a condition in which the squamous epithelium of the esophagus is replaced by columnar epithelium, a process called intestinal metaplasia. This condition normally occurs as a consequence of chronic acid exposure and has a predisposition for esophageal adenocarcinoma [14]. Biopsies of the esophagus are routinely taken to surveil Barrett's esophagus, and histologic diagnosis includes the presence or absence of dysplasia. Patients who have low- or high-grade dysplasia require endoscopic treatment in the form of ablative therapy to treat the abnormal tissue.

Radiofrequency ablation (RFA) uses radiofrequency energy to ablate Barrett's mucosa. This can be performed with the BARRX 360 (Medtronic, Minneapolis, MN, USA) circumferential device or one of many focal devices. The circumferential device is introduced over an endoscopically placed wire. The endoscope is advanced alongside this device. A balloon is then inflated up against Barrett's mucosa, and the radiofrequency energy is delivered. The radiofrequency energy generates a thermal injury to the tissue of limited thickness, essentially killing the dysplastic tissue so that it cannot progress to neoplasia [15]. The focal device works similarly but does not have a balloon. The device is attached to the end of the endoscope or passed through the endoscope channel. This is used for smaller areas of Barrett's mucosa with dysplasia. Endoscopic spray cryotherapy is a newer technique used in treating Barrett's mucosa. This method applies cold nitrogen or carbon dioxide gas via a device passed through the endoscope channel. The gas freezes Barrett's mucosa for approximately 40 s, again killing the dysplastic cells to prevent progression to neoplasia.

## Foreign Body Removal

Accidental foreign body or large food bolus ingestion can require endoscopic intervention under individual circumstances. Emergent indications for endoscopy include esophageal obstruction, sharp-pointed objects in the esophagus, and disk batteries in the esophagus. Urgent indications for endoscopy include dull objects in the esophagus, food impaction without esophageal obstruction, sharp-pointed objects in the stomach, magnets, and any objects larger than 6 cm in size. Typically, patients present with symptoms of dysphagia, odynophagia, inability to manage secretions, and pain in the neck, chest, or epigastric region.

Esophagogastroduodenoscopy can be performed for removal of foreign bodies. The endoscope is inserted into the esophagus, and once the foreign body is identified, several tools can be inserted through the endoscope channel and used to manage the foreign body. A rat-tooth forceps can be used, which contains three long, thin metal claws that open widely and closely tightly around objects. Once the object is engaged, the entire endoscope is removed with the rat-tooth forceps on the end holding the object. Similarly, there are alligator forceps which contain one flat forceps head and one angled forceps head to grab objects. Roth nets are snares with a net around the metal snare. They are opened around the foreign body and slowly closed, trapping the foreign body within the net. They too can then be removed by withdrawing the endoscope. Frequently, these maneuvers are performed repeatedly until the entire foreign body is removed. In the case of a food impaction, the food bolus can be pushed into the stomach lumen.

## Achalasia

Achalasia results from failure of relaxation of the lower esophageal sphincter (LES) associated with failed peristalsis of the lower esophagus. The etiology of primary achalasia is unclear, but secondary achalasia can occur from Chagas disease, amyloidosis, sarcoidosis, Sjogren syndrome, and eosinophilic esophagitis. Patients commonly present with complaints of dysphagia and regurgitation.

The treatment of achalasia is primarily directed at correcting the failure of the lower esophageal sphincter. Definitive treatment used to surgical myotomy. Endoscopic treatments include balloon dilation of the LES and botulinum toxin injection at the LES. These endoscopic treatments usually provide temporary relief. Peroral endoscopic myotomy (POEM) is a newer minimally invasive advanced endoscopic technique in which a myotomy of the lower esophageal sphincter is performed. This procedure includes making an incision in the esophageal mucosa, advancing the endoscope into the submucosa, and creating a tunnel through the submucosa extending to the gastric cardia. The muscularis propria is then cut with a needle-knife around the lower esophageal sphincter, correcting the persistent contraction of the sphincter. The main complications of this procedure include bleeding, infection, perforation, pneumomediastinum, pneumothorax, pneumoperitoneum, and GERD [16, 17]. POEM should only be carried out by a highly skilled therapeutic endoscopist or surgeon given high risk of complications. Multiple studies have shown that POEM is as effective as a laparoscopic Heller's myotomy (LHM) for achalasia with similar efficacy, length of hospital stay, and adverse events. Operative time appears to be shorter for POEM when compared to LHM.

# Stomach

## *Nutrition*

Failure to thrive, dysphagia, and malnutrition are common indications for placement of a percutaneous endoscopic gastrostomy (PEG) tube. An endoscope is advanced into the stomach, and the stomach is inflated with air. External finger pressure is applied, and a focal indentation of the gastric wall is seen endoscopically. The skin is cleansed with alcohol or povidone-iodine solution and anesthetized with lidocaine. A scalpel is used to make a horizontal incision in the skin, and a trocar is introduced into the stomach. A wire is advanced into the stomach. A snare, passed through the endoscope, is then used to grab the wire, and the whole endoscope is removed from the patient with the wire pulled out of the mouth. The PEG tube is secured to the wire, and the wire is pulled from the abdominal wall to pull the PEG tube through the mouth and into the stomach. The PEG tube bumper is pulled up snugly to the stomach wall. It is then cut to the appropriate length and clamped. In order to prevent peristomal infection, a dose of antibiotics is given prior to this procedure. A jejunal extension tube can be placed through the PEG tube and advanced under fluoroscopy or by endoscopy to the jejunum, when jejunal feeding and gastric venting are required. This is often referred to as a PEG-J tube. Percutaneous endoscopic jejunostomy (PEJ) tube placement, where a feeding tube is directly placed into the jejunum, can also be performed. This is done when jejunal feeding is required and/or when gastric feeding is not possible.

## *Endobariatrics*

Obesity is a worldwide epidemic, and new therapies are continually being developed to help patients with weight loss. Endobariatrics is a growing field of minimally invasive endoscopic procedures implemented to aid patients with weight loss. Intragastric balloon therapy is a technique in which a soft, saline-filled balloon is inserted into the stomach to stimulate the sensation of satiety and reduce food consumption. This procedure is indicated for patients with a body mass index (BMI) of 30–35, for patients with a BMI 40 or greater who choose to not undergo bariatric surgery, or for patients with a BMI greater than 50 to be used as a bridge to bariatric surgery. These balloons can be kept in place for 6 months and then need to be removed [18]. Endoscopic sleeve gastroplasty (ESG) is another approach to bariatric therapy in which the stomach is endoscopically sutured, narrowing the lumen and reducing the total volume similar to a surgical sleeve gastrectomy. This is mechanistically restrictive to achieve weight loss. One study by Sharaiha et al. demonstrated a 20.9% loss of total body weight at 2-year follow-up [19].

# Biliary

Endoscopic retrograde cholangiopancreatography (ERCP) is an advanced technique that incorporates both endoscopy and fluoroscopy to closely examine and treat conditions of the biliary tree, gallbladder, and pancreas. Major indications for ERCP include the diagnosis and decompression of biliary obstruction. Etiologies of biliary obstruction include choledocholithiasis, benign strictures, and malignant strictures (i.e., pancreatic malignancy or cholangiocarcinoma). In this regard, ERCP is not only used for diagnostic purposes but also is therapeutic for decompressing the pancreaticobiliary system and alleviating the obstruction to permit bile and pancreatic enzyme flow.

The endoscope used in ERCP is a side-viewing duodenoscope which is blindly inserted through the esophagus and stomach to reach the second portion of the duodenum to access the biliopancreatic ampulla (also known as the ampulla of Vater). The ampulla is the junction at which the common bile duct (CBD) and the ventral pancreatic duct (PD) meet. A wire is then used to cannulate either duct depending on the indication. After the wire is inserted, contrast dye is then injected which can be visualized under fluoroscopy to view either the biliary ducts (cholangiogram) or the pancreatic ducts (pancreatogram). This enables the endoscopist to visualize the abnormality and intervene with specialized accessory tools to cut, dilate, and obtain tissue samples or stent the affected area. ERCP is associated with a 5–7% risk of pancreatitis. Less common risks include bleeding, infection, or perforation.

## *Choledocholithiasis*

The first-line management for choledocholithiasis is ERCP with sphincterotomy and stone extraction. If one or more stones are identified in the CBD, stone removal can be performed with balloon extraction or with a stone basket. If these methods are unsuccessful, more advanced methods can be attempted, such as pneumatic balloon dilation, mechanical lithotripsy, or laser lithotripsy [20].

This procedure begins with advancing the duodenoscope into the second portion of the duodenum and positioning the duodenoscope over the ampulla, the entrance to the CBD. Cannulation of the ampulla is performed with a sphincterotome, a device that permits cannulation and passage of a guidewire. Once the guidewire is in the CBD, dye is injected to view the location of stones via fluoroscopy.

Sphincterotomy, which refers to cutting of the biliary sphincter, enlarging the opening, and permitting stones to pass, is then performed. If sphincterotomy is insufficient in removing all stones or if larger stones are present, then a balloon dilator is inserted into the CBD to expand the duct and sweep the entire duct for additional stone and sludge removal. Depending on the presence or absence of additional stones in the CBD or gallbladder, a stent may be placed into the CBD to prevent recurrence or prevent cholangitis. These stents are normally plastic and remain in place for 2–3 months before being removed with a subsequent procedure.

## Biliary Strictures

Strictures of the pancreaticobiliary tree, both benign and malignant, can cause symptomatic obstruction causing jaundice, cholangitis, or pancreatitis. Endoscopic therapy includes identification of the stricture via fluoroscopy, decompression via sphincterotomy, and subsequent catheter dilation or balloon dilation if the stricture is tight. The duodenoscope is advanced to the ampulla in the second portion of the duodenum. The guidewire is then used to cannulate the CBD. Dye is injected and fluoroscopy is used to identify the stricture and likely upstream biliary ductal dilation. An additional device is inserted via another channel in the duodenoscope to obtain brushings of the stricture for histological evaluation. A plastic or metal stent is then advanced over the guidewire and deployed at the site of the stricture to allow bile flow. The stent is then removed subsequently if the stricture heals or stent exchange is performed in the case of persistent or malignant strictures. Metal stents are usually used instead of plastic stents in the setting of surgically unresectable malignancy. There is some data suggesting fully covered metal stents, which are removable, can be used in benign strictures as well, decreasing the total number of ERCPs and possible procedure-related complications to reach stricture resolution [21].

Cholangiocarcinoma is a cancer that originated from the bile duct epithelium. It presents oftentimes with jaundice due to biliary obstruction. Cholangiocarcinoma involving the liver hilum, also known as a Klatskin tumor, is oftentimes surgically unresectable. In these situations, photodynamic therapy (PDT) delivered via ERCP has been shown to prolong survival, improve biliary drainage, and improve quality of life. In one study survival was prolonged from 98 to 493 days [22]. Radiofrequency ablation (RFA) is another modality that can be offered endoscopically for patients with unresectable hilar cholangiocarcinoma. [23] PDT and RFA are offered at few highly specialized tertiary care hospitals in the United States.

## Bile Leak

A bile leak is a possible complication occurring postoperatively in gallbladder or biliary surgeries. Standard treatment for a bile leak is ERCP with placement of a temporary bile duct stent. This procedure begins with standard technique of duodenoscope insertion and identification of the ampulla. The guidewire is inserted through the ampulla into the common bile duct and passed the region of the surgical anastomosis. The sphincterotome is passed over the guidewire and dye is injected. Fluoroscopy is then used to identify the site of the leak. Sphincterotomy is performed to decompress and improve outflow of bile. A temporary plastic stent is then advanced over the guide wire into the bile duct. The goal is for bile to flow via the path of least resistance, which in this case would now be into the duodenum. The stent is left in place until healing of the leak is completed and removed thereafter.

## Cholangioscopy and Pancreatoscopy

Cholangioscopy and pancreatoscopy are endoscopic methods for direct visualization of the bile ducts and pancreatic duct, respectively. Common indications for this diagnostic and therapeutic procedure include treatment of intrahepatic biliary stones, identifying and better characterizing benign vs malignant biliary strictures, and identifying biliary tumors [24]. This procedure is always performed in conjunction with ERCP. This procedure begins with standard duodenoscope insertion to the second portion of the duodenum where the ampulla is situated. Cannulation of the CBD is performed, and a guidewire is introduced with confirmation of position in the CBD via fluoroscopy. The cholangioscope, which is a smaller catheter with an optical probe tip, is then inserted into a channel of the duodenoscope. The cholangioscope is then advanced passed the duodenoscope for direct visualization of the bile ducts. If a stone is identified, catheter-directed electrohydraulic or laser lithotripsy is performed. If a stricture is identified, a special forceps can be introduced for obtaining biopsies. Cholangioscopy and pancreatoscopy can be utilized for mapping of pancreaticobiliary malignancies and can potentially alter surgical resection plans [25].

## Pancreas

### Pancreatic Cysts

Endoscopic ultrasound (EUS), either alone or with fine needle aspiration, is widely used in the diagnostic workup of various pancreatic cystic lesions. In comparison to other imaging modalities, EUS allows high-resolution imaging of pancreatic lesions and their characteristics. EUS has the added benefit of fine needle aspiration (FNA), where under real-time ultrasound guidance, a needle is advanced into these lesions for both diagnostic and therapeutic purposes. In this way, EUS-FNA can safely aspirate cystic contents and biopsy the cyst wall or nodules within the cyst. The aspirates obtained can be analyzed for enzymes, cytology, tumor markers, and DNA analysis, thereby helping to distinguish between malignant and benign lesions [26]. Furthermore, EUS-FNA is often used in the perioperative period in the evaluation of malignant solid and cystic lesions for staging and diagnosis. EUS can delineate malignant cyst size, the presence of lymphadenopathy, vasculature involvement, and the presence of nearby organ metastasis.

Many different types of cysts are amenable to endoscopic drainage and decompression with the main limiting factor being the presence of an accessible, matured wall. Walled-off pancreatic fluid collections normally result from pancreatitis, trauma, or prior surgical procedures. Endoscopic cystogastrostomy is a minimally invasive procedure frequently performed in unresolving, symptomatic pancreatic pseudocysts or in walled-off pancreatic necrosis that is amenable to drainage [27]. These cysts are identified by a bulge in the gastric lumen or with endoscopic ultrasound. Electrocautery is used to make an incision, followed by advancement of a guidewire into the fluid collection over which a balloon dilator is used to widen the tract. Finally, a temporary stent is placed, and its position is confirmed using endosonography or fluoroscopy. With the advent of lumen-apposing metal stents (LAMS), the stent can be advanced directly into the cystic cavity using electrocautery and then deployed under endoscopic, endosonographic, and fluoroscopic visualization. These cautery-enhanced LAMS drastically decrease procedure time [28].

## Chronic Pancreatitis

A common complication of chronic pancreatitis leading to recurrent hospitalization is pain. Pain in chronic pancreatitis often stems from increased pressure in the main pancreatic duct (PD) from outflow obstruction. Etiologies for obstruction include intrapancreatic conditions such PD strictures, PD stones, sphincter stenosis, pancreatic cancer, or extra-pancreatic conditions such as biliary and duodenal obstruction. Recurrent pancreatitis leads to peripancreatic and celiac neuronal inflammation which manifests as chronic pain, often persisting even after the pancreatitis resolves. The nerve fibers that run through the pancreas join the celiac plexus which lies just anterior to the aorta. These nerve root ganglions can be accessed by EUS-FNA for treatment of this chronic pain. Celiac plexus block is a minimally invasive endoscopic procedure in which the celiac nerve root ganglion is injected with an anesthetic and steroid medication. The celiac plexus is first identified with the EUS endoscope by identifying the celiac axis. Then, a needle is advanced through the endoscope channel onto this region, and the medications are delivered. This normally provides immediate pain relief, although the lasting effects are variable and the procedure is frequently repeated. Celiac plexus neurolysis is a similar procedure; however, the celiac nerve root ganglion is injected with an alcohol. This obliterates the nerve ending and is normally only indicated for unresectable pancreatic cancer given long-term complications including retroperitoneal fibrosis.

## *Necrotizing Pancreatitis and Endoscopic Necrosectomy*

Necrotizing pancreatitis is a complication that is seen in a small percentage of patients with acute pancreatitis that do not clinically improve with standard medical management. Necrotizing pancreatitis can lead to sterile or infected walled-off necrosis. Endoscopic drainage and necrosectomy, the removal of the necrotic debris, is often indicated, especially in instances of mechanical obstruction, persistent abdominal symptoms, and progression to sepsis. The standard approach is to visualize the necrotic collection endosonographically in relation to the adjacent stomach or duodenum, puncturing the collection and forming a tract with balloon dilation. This can also be done using the cautery-enhanced LAMS, as mentioned previously. The collection is then accessed with various accessory tools including snares, forceps, irrigation devices, and baskets. The tissue is debrided and removed, and the temporary stent is left in place permitting drainage of the remaining cystic contents into the stomach or duodenum. Based on the size of the necrotic collection, this procedure may be repeated multiple times in order to completely remove all of the necrosis. The main benefits of this approach include the lack of incisions which limits wound infections and being a targeted approach to limit spread of the infection preventing a systemic inflammatory response. These translate into improved healing rates and better tolerability [29]. Endoscopic necrosectomy has been shown to reduce morbidity when compared to surgical necrosectomy.

## Conclusion

The field of endoscopy continues to grow as technology advances. Gastroenterology, specifically advanced endoscopy, and minimally invasive surgery will continue to converge as newer techniques and procedures are envisioned. This will revolutionize care for patients. Therapeutic endosonography and endoscopic surgery are at the forefront of this revolution in gastroenterology. EUS is now being used to drain gallbladders in patients that are not surgical candidates for cholecystectomy [28, 30]. EUS has also been used to perform endoscopic gastrojejunostomy for patients with malignant gastric outlet obstruction [31]. Endoscopic full-thickness resection is being carried out for localized tumors of the GI tract [32]. Endoscopy will continue to evolve and progress, which will offer patients truly minimally invasive options for certain gastrointestinal conditions.

## References

1. Laine L, Jensen DM. Management of patients with ulcer bleeding. Am J Gastroenterol. 2012;107:345–60.
2. Laine L, McQuaid KR. Endoscopic therapy for bleeding ulcers: an evidence-based approach based on meta-analyses of randomized controlled trials. Clin Gastroenterol Hepatol. 2009;7:33–47.

3. Kwan V, Bourke MJ, Williams SJ, et al. Argon plasma coagulation in the management of symptomatic gastrointestinal vascular lesions: experience in 100 consecutive patients with long-term follow-up. Am J Gastroenterol. 2006;101(1):58–63.
4. Hwang JH, Shergill AK, Acosta RD, et al. The role of endoscopy in the management of variceal hemorrhage. Gastrointest Endosc. 2014;80(2):221–7.
5. Bhat YM, Weilert F, Fredrick RT, et al. EUS-guided treatment of gastric fundal varices with combined injection of coils and cyanoacrylate glue: a large U.S. experience over 6 years. Gastrointest Endosc. 2016;83(6):1164–72.
6. Kantsevoy SV, Bitner M. Nonsurgical treatment of actively bleeding internal hemorrhoids with a novel endoscopic device (with video). Gastrointest Endosc. 2013;78(4):649–53.
7. Jensen DM, Machicado GA, Jutabha R, et al. Urgent colonoscopy for the diagnosis and treatment of severe diverticular hemorrhage. N Engl J Med. 2000;342(2):78–82.
8. Akerman PA. Spiral enteroscopy versus double-balloon enteroscopy: choosing the right tool for the job. Gastrointest Endosc. 2013;77(2):252–4.
9. Kaltenbach T, Soetikno R. Endoscopic resection of large colon polyps. Gastrointest Endosc Clin N Am. 2013;23(1):137–52.
10. Holmes I, Friedland S. Endoscopic mucosal resection versus endoscopic submucosal dissection for large polyps: a western Colonoscopist's view. Clin Endosc. 2016;49(5):454–6.
11. Varadarajulu S, Banerjee S, Barth B, et al. Enteral stents. Gastrointest Endosc. 2011;74(3):455–64.
12. Katz PO, Gerson LB, Vela MF, et al. Diagnosis and management of gastroesophageal reflux disease. Am J Gastroenterol. 2013;108:308–28.
13. Trad KS, Fox MA, Simoni G. Transoral fundoplication offers durable symptom control for chronic GERD: 3-year report from the TEMPO randomized trial with a crossover arm. Surg Endosc. 2016;31:2498–508.
14. Shaheen NJ, Falk GW, Iyer PG, et al. Diagnosis and management of barrett's esophagus. Am J Gastroenterol. 2016;111:30–50.
15. Shaheen NJ, Sharma P, Overholt BF, et al. Radiofrequency ablation in Barrett's esophagus with dysplasia. N Engl J Med. 2009;360:2277–88.
16. Inoue H, Minami H, Kobayashi Y, et al. Peroral endoscopic myotomy (POEM) for esophageal achalasia. Endoscopy. 2010;42(4):265–71.
17. Talukdar R, Inoue H, Reddy DN. Efficacy of peroral endoscopic myotomy (POEM) in the treatment of achalasia: a systematic review and meta-analysis. Surg Endosc. 2015;29:3030.
18. Pickett-Blakely O, Newberry C. Future therapies in obesity. Gastroenterol Clin N Am. 2016;45(4):705–14.
19. Sharaiha RZ, Kumta NA, Saumoy M, et al. Endoscopic sleeve gastroplasty significantly reduces body mass index and metabolic complications in obese patients. Clin Gastroenterol Hepatol. 2017;15(4):504–10.
20. Maple JT, Ikenberry SO, Anderson MA, et al. The role of endoscopy in the management of choledocholithiasis. Gastrointest Endosc. 2011;74(4):731–44.
21. Cote G, Slivka A, Tarnasky P, et al. Effect of covered metallic stents compared with plastic stents on benign biliary stricture resolution: a randomized clinical trial. JAMA. 2016;315(12):1250–7.
22. Ortner ME, Caca K, Berr F, et al. Successful photodynamic therapy for nonresectable cholangiocarcinoma: a randomized prospective study. Gastroenterology. 2003;125(5):1355–63.
23. Figueroa-Barjoas P, Bakhru M, Habib N, et al. Safety and efficacy of radiofrequency ablation in the management of unresectable bile duct and pancreatic cancer: a novel palliation technique. J Oncol. 2013;2013:910897.
24. Komanduri S, Thosani N, Abu Dayyeh BK, et al. Cholangiopancreatoscopy. Gastrointest Endosc. 2016;84(2):209–21.
25. Tyberg A, Raijman I, Siddiqui A, et al. Digital pancreatic cholangioscopy for mapping of pancreaticobiliary neoplasia: can we alter the surgical resection margin? J Clin Gastroenterol. 2018 Mar 6. [Epub ahead of print].

26. Polkowski M, Jenssen C, Kaye P, et al. Technical aspects of endoscopic ultrasound (EUS)-guided sampling in gastroenterology: European society of gastrointestinal endoscopy (ESGE) technical guidelines-March 2017. Endoscopy. 2017;49:989–1006.
27. Muthusamy VR, Chandrasekhara V, Acosta RD, et al. The role of endoscopy in the diagnosis and treatment of inflammatory pancreatic fluid collections. Gastrointest Endosc. 2016;83(3):481–8.
28. Itoi T, Binmoeller KF, Shah J, et al. Clinical evaluation of a novel lumen-apposing metal stent for endosonography-guided pancreatic pseudocyst and gallbladder drainage. Gastrointest Endosc. 2012;75(4):870–6.
29. Bakker OJ, van Santvoort HC, et al. Endoscopic transgastric vs surgical necrosectomy for infected necrotizing pancreatitis: a randomized trial. JAMA. 2012;307(10):1053–61.
30. Xu M, Kahaleh M. EUS-guided transmural gallbladder drainage: a new era has begun. Therap Adv Gastroenterol. 2016;9(2):138–40.
31. Tyberg A, Perez-Miranda M, et al. Endoscopic ultrasound-guided gastrojejunostomy with a lumen-apposing metal stent: a multicenter, international experience. Endosc Int Open. 2016;4(3):E276–81.
32. Vitali F, Naegel A, Siebler J, et al. Endoscopic full-thickness resection with an over-the-scope clip device (FTRD) in the colorectum: results from a university tertiary referral center. Endosc Int Open. 2018;6(1):E98–E103.

# Chapter 3
# Benign Esophageal Disease

**Keith King, Rachel E. NeMoyer, and Susannah Wise**

## Introduction

Benign esophageal disease comprises many different diseases and disease pathology including gastroesophageal reflux disease (GERD), hiatal hernia, and achalasia.

GERD is an all-encompassing term used to describe people who have symptoms of reflux disease, but do not necessarily have esophageal inflammation or esophageal damage. A subset of GERD includes reflux esophagitis, which is defined as having histologic or endoscopic evidence of esophageal inflammation [1]. If GERD is left untreated, up to 30% of patients will have evidence of esophageal damage on endoscopy [2]. Due to the broad spectrum of symptoms and conditions described as reflux, no consensus exists for the definition of typical reflux disease [3]. The Montreal Working Group describes troublesome reflux if a person has mild symptoms occurring 2 or more days a week or if moderate/severe symptoms occur greater than 1 day per week [3]. Limitations exist when describing the prevalence of GERD; however, it has been stated that GERD may affect nearly two thirds of adults in the USA at some point in their life, which equates to a significant public health problem [4, 5].

K. King (✉)
General Surgery, Rutgers Robert Wood Johnson Medical School, New Brunswick, NJ, USA

R. E. NeMoyer · S. Wise
Rutgers Robert Wood Johnson Medical School, New Brunswick, NJ, USA
e-mail: ssw1x@rwjms.rutgers.edu

© Springer Nature Switzerland AG 2019
C. Rezac, K. Donohue (eds.), *The Internist's Guide to Minimally Invasive Gastrointestinal Surgery*, Clinical Gastroenterology,
https://doi.org/10.1007/978-3-319-96631-1_3

Hiatal hernias have been classified into five different subtypes (I–IV) depending on anatomical considerations [6].

(a) Type I: Sliding hernias, where the GE junction moves above the diaphragm with the stomach remaining in its usual alignment [7, 8]
(b) Type II: Pure paraesophageal hernias where the GE junction remains in its usual anatomic position, but a portion of fundus herniates through the diaphragm hiatus
(c) Type III: Combination of type I and II with the GE junction and the fundus herniating through the diaphragmatic hiatus
(d) Type IV: Herniation of another structure other than the stomach, such as the colon or omentum within the hernia sac

The majority of hiatal hernias (>95%) are type I [9]. The incidence of hiatal hernias increases with age, with approximately 60% of people age 50 or greater having a hiatal hernia [10].

Finally, achalasia is a rare motility disorder of the esophagus that is defined as the absence of esophageal peristalsis and incomplete relaxation of the lower esophageal sphincter (LES) when swallowing [11]. Achalasia is rare and has an incidence of 1.6 cases per 100,000 individuals per year, with men and women being affected equally [12]. The usual age of diagnosis is between ages 25 and 60 [12].

## Patient Presentation

Patients presenting with benign esophageal disease may have similar initial symptoms. The most common symptoms of patients presenting to the primary care doctor include heartburn, dysphagia for solids and/or liquids, regurgitation, chest pain, cough, hoarseness, voice change, and/or weight loss [13]. To help differentiate the possible cause of the symptoms, a careful history is essential to determine severity, length of symptoms, and timing of symptoms. A physical exam is warranted to exclude other causes of these presenting symptoms; however, diagnosing esophageal disease requires further testing for confirmation [14].

## Work-Up/Diagnosis

Currently there is no agreement as to which studies and in which order should be obtained for the diagnosis of GERD; however, many believe that an endoscopy should be one of the initial studies [15]. To assess the diagnosis of GERD, many studies are available that can give objective documentation of this diagnosis. Upper endoscopy/esophagogastroduodenoscopy (EGD) is usually an early tool to aid in diagnosis. On endoscopy, "mucosal breaks" may be visualized which are areas of erythema or slough that are clearly separate and demarcated from adjacent normal-looking mucosa [16]. Biopsies should be taken from any areas with suspected changes such as metaplasia or dysplasia [17]. Evaluation for Barrett's esophagus is important. Additionally, cancer needs to be excluded as a cause of symptoms.

If endoscopy fails to show pathological evidence of reflux, another test to diagnose reflux is a 24-hour esophageal ph-metry. This involves a thin-tube device to be inserted down a patient's nose, terminating about 2 inches above the LES. More recently, pH evaluation is done using a Bravo capsule clipped endoscopically to the esophageal mucosa. This is a more appealing alternative to a tube coming out of the nose. The capsule releases on its own after a short period of time and is eliminated thru the GI tract [17]. Esophageal manometry is another alternative diagnostic tool used. This is commonly obtained prior to surgery to help identify any conditions that may contraindicate fundoplication; however, this study is not required and is usually up to surgeon discretion [18, 19]. Finally, a barium swallow may be obtained to further define the anatomy. This is especially useful in patients with enlarged hiatal hernias or a shortened esophagus [17].

To diagnose and delineate hiatal hernias, multiple diagnostic options are available. A simple first step is to obtain a plain chest radiograph. This may identify soft tissue densities with air-fluid levels within the chest, indicating a possible hiatal hernia. Specific loops of bowel may be seen within the chest and lead to a diagnosis of hiatal hernia [20]. Contrast studies such as a barium swallow, as discussed earlier in the GERD section, may help to gauge the size of the hernia and/or locate the GE junction related to the hiatus. These studies may also help identify a short esophagus, again important in preoperative planning [21]. Real-time video swallow studies may also help identify transit time and bolus transport issues. Due to high risk of aspiration with a hiatal hernia, water-soluble contrast material, such as gastrografin should be avoided due to risk of aspiration pneumonitis, with barium being the preferred contrast material [22]. CT scans may be of use in the acute setting to diagnose complications related to hiatal and paraesophageal hernias. On CT, one may see air-fluid levels within the chest, and the GE junction may be noted to be cephalad to its normal anatomical position [23]. An EGD may be performed as well, although this is not always necessary for diagnosis or treatment. In the emergency setting, EGD may be helpful in assessing gastric viability in an acutely incarcerated hernia or volvulus.

Esophageal manometry may be used in conjunction with a pH probe when concerned for concomitant hiatal hernia and reflux disease. In patients with a sliding hiatal hernia, it may be difficult to accurately place the pH probe without esophageal manometry guidance. Manometry may also help locate the level of the diaphragmatic crura and the location of the LES [24].

Diagnosis of achalasia should be confirmed with a barium swallow/esophagram. A "bird's beak" appearance or a smooth tapering of the lower esophagus leading to a closed LES will be seen on a positive study. Manometry can also be used to diagnose achalasia by showing aperistalsis and incomplete or insufficient LES relaxation when swallowing. Finally, patients should undergo EGD to exclude other causes of aperistalsis such as a tumor at the GE junction [25].

# Hiatal Hernia

## *Indications for Surgery*

Although most hiatal hernias can be managed medically, laparoscopic hiatal hernia repair can benefit some patients with symptomatic hiatal hernias. For asymptomatic type I hernias, surgery is not recommended [26]. However, surgery may be of benefit to patients with type I hernias who have complications of GERD such as strictures, ulcers, bleeding, or pulmonary complications such as asthma, recurrent aspiration pneumonia, or chronic cough [27]. In these patients, GERD, not the sliding hernia, is the indication for surgery, and a fundoplication must be performed [28].

Symptomatic or complicated paraesophageal hernias should be surgically repaired as a significant proportion of this type of hiatal hernia can become incarcerated or possibly result in gastric volvulus leading to gastric perforation. The timing of repair of paraesophageal hernias depends on the presentation. Acute gastric volvulus, uncontrolled bleeding, obstruction, strangulation, perforation, or severe respiratory compromise secondary to mass effect of the hernia requires emergent repair. More commonly, paraesophageal hernias present with symptoms such as refractory GERD, dysphagia, early satiety, postprandial chest pain, or vomiting can be repaired electively [29]. Completely asymptomatic paraesophageal hernias do not always necessitate surgical repair. The patient's age and comorbidities should be weighed with the risks of surgery in evaluating whether to proceed with repairing asymptomatic paraesophageal hernias.

## *Operation*

Hiatal hernia repair can be performed through the chest or the abdomen and can be approached using minimally invasive techniques or traditional open surgery. The morbidity of this surgery is significantly reduced when using a laparoscopic approach when compared to open surgery [30]. Laparoscopic surgery has been shown to be as effective as the open approach in reducing recurrences. With consideration to the similar efficacy combined with decreased perioperative morbidity, laparoscopy or robotic-assisted techniques have become the preferred method for repairing hiatal hernias.

Surgery involves dissecting out and reducing the hernia and its contents into the abdomen, closing the hiatal defect, and finally performing an antireflux procedure. In order to prevent recurrence of the hiatal hernia, the hernia sac must be completely dissected from the mediastinal structures and excised if possible [31]. Next, the lower esophagus must be mobilized sufficiently to allow the gastroesophageal (GE) junction to return to the abdomen. If the esophagus cannot be adequately mobilized, a neo-esophagus can be created from the stomach using an esophageal lengthening technique known as a Collis gastroplasty [32].

After reduction and excision of the hernia sac, the hiatal defect must be closed. The crura of the diaphragm are closed inferiorly and posteriorly to the esophagus either with a primary suture repair or with the addition of mesh reinforcement. Several randomized controlled studies have demonstrated that mesh reinforcement during hiatal hernia repair may lead to a decreased short-term recurrence rate [33–35]. However, there is insufficient evidence regarding the long-term benefit of mesh reinforcement. When making the decision to use mesh, consideration must be given to serious mesh-related complications such as mesh erosion, esophageal stenosis, and the need for reoperation. Given these potential complications, using biologic mesh is generally preferred to using synthetic mesh.

Once the hiatal defect is closed, performing a fundoplication is beneficial in treating reflux and decreasing recurrence rates of the hernia. Both complete (Nissen) and partial fundoplications can reestablish competency of the gastroesophageal sphincter and are a necessary component of treating type I sliding hernias [24]. However, fundoplication may increase postoperative dysphagia, and thus routine fundoplication is not necessarily beneficial to all patients [36].

An ideal hiatal hernia repair results in the permanent retention of the stomach and GE junction within the abdomen. Fixing the stomach to the abdominal wall with an anterior gastropexy may help decrease rates of recurrence when combined with primary repair of the hiatal hernia [37]. Anterior gastropexy can be accomplished with either sutures or with a gastrostomy tube. The use of a gastrostomy tube may additionally facilitate postoperative care in select patients such as those with delayed gastric emptying. Endoscopic reduction of hiatal hernias combined with percutaneous endoscopic gastrostomy (PEG) tube placement without primary repair is an option in extremely high-risk patients. However, significantly higher recurrence rates are associated with this procedure, and primary repair is preferred [38].

## Postoperative Management

After minimally invasive hiatal hernia repair, patients are admitted to the hospital and kept on antiemetics to minimize nausea and vomiting which could potentially disrupt the hernia repair resulting in early recurrence. In asymptomatic patients, it is not necessary to perform routine postoperative contrast studies. Early postoperative dysphagia is common occurring in up to 50% of patients. The patient's diet should be advanced slowly from clear liquids to solids. It is important to pay close attention to the patient's nutritional status and caloric intake given the frequency of postoperative dysphagia. Although some weight loss after minimally invasive hiatal hernia repair is normal, weight loss in excess of 20 lbs. (9 kg) should prompt further evaluation and possibly intervention for dysphagia [29].

The mortality and morbidity of elective minimally invasive hiatal hernia repair are relatively low with 30-day mortality rates ranging from 0.8% to 1.7% [39, 40]. The morbidity and mortality significantly increase in emergent hiatal hernia repair.

Most common complications of hiatal repair are pneumonia (4.0%), pulmonary embolism (3.4%), heart failure (2.6%), and postoperative leak (2.5%) [39].

One of the most important long-term complications of minimally invasive hiatal hernia repair is recurrence of the hernia. The rate of radiographic recurrence is generally higher than the clinical recurrence of symptoms and rarely requires reoperation. Rathore et al. reported in a meta-analysis a clinical recurrence rate of 10.2% and a radiographic recurrence rate of 25% [41]. Reoperation for hiatal hernias is technically challenging and should be reserved for patients with severe recurrent symptoms.

## Gastroesophageal Reflux Disease (GERD)

### Indications for Surgery

Surgery for reflux is generally reserved for patients with complications of reflux or the inability or unwillingness to take lifelong medication. When the diagnosis of GERD has been confirmed, surgery should be considered in patients:

1. With persistent symptoms despite optimal medical management
2. With well-controlled GERD who wish for a onetime, definitive treatment
3. Who have complications of GERD such as Barrett's esophagus or peptic stricture [42]
4. Who have extraesophageal manifestations of GERD including:

    (a) Respiratory manifestations such as cough, wheezing, or aspiration
    (b) Ear, nose, and throat manifestations such as hoarseness, sore throat, or otitis media
    (c) Dental manifestations such as enamel erosion

5. Who are unable to tolerate or afford lifetime medication

The role of surgical intervention for patients with symptoms of asthma related to reflux has not been clearly defined, but some studies have suggested that surgery may improve asthma symptoms, asthma medication use, and pulmonary function [43].

If Barrett's esophagus is suspected when upper endoscopy is performed during the preoperative assesment of GERD, four quadrant biopsies are taken to confirm the diagnosis and assess the histological grade. Endoscopic mucosal resection (EMR) can be used at this time to resect areas of ulceration and nodularity to rule out the presence of neoplasia. If adenocarcinoma involving the submucosa and deeper is detected, the patient is not a candidate for antireflux surgery and should be referred for radiation, chemotherapy, and possible esophagectomy [28]. High-grade intraepithelial neoplasia (HGIN) and intramucosal carcinoma (IMC) can by treated with endoscopic techniques such as photodynamic therapy (PDT), EMR, and radiofrequency ablation (RFA). When these techniques accomplish complete histological eradication, then antireflux surgery may be considered [44]. If biopsy demonstrates nonneoplastic intestinal metaplasia (IM), indefinite for neoplasia (IND), or low-grade intraepithelial neoplasia (LGIN), then antireflux surgery can be offered without prior endoscopic eradication [45].

## *Operation*

Multiple factors such as the degree of esophageal shortening, disturbances of esophageal motility, prior operations, and expertise in laparoscopic techniques play a role in deciding the optimal approach for patients undergoing antireflux surgery. When comparing a laparoscopic minimally invasive approach with open surgery, multiple randomized controlled studies have demonstrated that the laparoscopic approach is associated with shorter hospital stays, earlier return to work, and less complications in the short term. Long-term failure rates of both the laparoscopic and open approaches were similar. Laparoscopy, however, was associated with longer operative times and higher rates of reoperation when compared to open surgery [28].

Multiple antireflux procedures have been described in the treatment of GERD. The goal of these procedures is generally to recreate a functional lower esophageal sphincter. The Nissen fundoplication is the most commonly performed antireflux surgery and results in a 90% symptomatic improvement [46]. Laparoscopic Nissen fundoplication is performed under general anesthesia using five small (5–12 mm) incisions. First, the fundus of the stomach and distal esophagus are completely mobilized. The short gastric vessels are only divided if further mobility is needed to create the wrap [47, 48]. If a hiatal hernia is encountered, it is dissected and reduced into the abdomen followed by narrowing of the esophageal hiatus through crural closure. Biologic mesh reinforcement should be considered if the hiatal defect is large [28]. Finally, fundoplication is performed by suturing the posterior and anterior walls of the gastric fundus anteriorly together around an intraesophageal dilator to create a 360° wrap.

Although laparoscopic Nissen fundoplication is the most commonly performed antireflux procedure, a number of alternatives and modifications exist and may be appropriate in various settings. A partial 270° wrap (Toupet) can be used in patients with severe motor abnormalities [49]. However, a tailored approach to esophageal motility is unwarranted as esophageal motility generally improves as symptoms of GERD are controlled [28]. Other antireflux options include an anterior 180° wrap (Dor), transthoracic partial fundoplication (Bell Mark IV), and imbricating the lesser curve of the stomach around the esophagus and then tethering this complex to the median arcuate ligament (Hill gastropexy). When compared to the traditional 360° wrap, partial fundoplication is associated with less postoperative dysphagia, fewer reoperations, and a similar effectiveness in controlling symptoms of GERD [28]. Anterior wraps are generally associated with less postoperative dysphagia [50] but are less effective in reflux control [51]. In morbidly obese patients with a BMI greater than 35, gastric bypass should be used as the treatment of GERD because of the high failure rates of fundoplication in this population [52].

## *Postoperative Management*

After undergoing a minimally invasive Nissen fundoplication, patients are admitted to the hospital and started on a liquid diet. The management of these patients in the postoperative period depends on the symptoms related to the size and tightness of the wrap. Perioperative and early postoperative dysphagia is one of the most common complications of Nissen fundoplication with rates reported as high as 76% [53]. However, most studies show dysphagia rates to be less than 20% at 1 year [28]. Generally, dysphagia is managed with dietary modification and a continued liquid diet. However, dysphagia that persists more than 12 weeks should prompt further evaluation. Approximately 6–12% of patients who undergo Nissen fundoplication will require endoscopic dilatation [54]. Patients with a 360° wrap may be candidates for conversion to a partial wrap to relieve symptoms of persistent dysphagia.

Other complications specific to minimally invasive antireflux surgery include gastric or esophageal perforation and pneumothorax. Severe pain, intractable emesis, fever, tachycardia, or leukocytosis in the immediate postoperative period should prompt an evaluation for perforated viscous. The rate of gastric and esophageal perforation is related to the technique used and surgical experience and ranges from 0% to 4% with the higher rates reported in redo fundoplication [28]. Pneumothorax has been reported in 0–1.5% of cases and is likely related to excessive hiatal dissection.

One late postoperative complication associated with Nissen fundoplication is gas bloat syndrome, or the sensation of intestinal gas with the inability to belch. Although the etiology is not clearly understood, this syndrome may be related to delayed gastric emptying, aerophagia, or vagal dysfunction. Mild symptoms can be managed by avoiding carbonated beverages, simethicone, or metoclopramide. Pyloroplasty, pyloric botox, and pneumatic pyloric dilatation can be offered in select patients with severe persistent symptoms [55].

Antireflux surgery can be performed with minimal morbidity and mortality and effectively improves LES pressure and decreases acid reflux leading to high patient satisfaction rates and improved quality of life. Most studies report greater than 90% satisfaction with results after laparoscopic fundoplication. The continued use of acid-reducing medications after antireflux is generally reported as less than 20% [56]. Antireflux surgery is most effective in treating typical symptoms of GERD, while atypical symptoms such pulmonary symptoms, although they mostly improve, have a higher rate of persistence [28].

## Achalasia

### *Indications for Surgery*

The goal of treatment for achalasia is to improve patient's symptoms by decreasing the pressure of the LES in hopes of minimizing the functional obstruction

[2]. Treatment is pertinent when achalasia is suspected and diagnosed. A dilated esophagus with severely limited bolus transit time can occur with treatment delay, which can lead to perforation and/or aspiration [57]. Early diagnosis and prompt treatment of achalasia is essential in preventing any of the end-stage outcomes.

Various treatment options exist initially to treat achalasia including pharmcological interventions (oral nitrates, calcium channel blockers, or botulinum injections), pneumatic dilation, peroral endoscopic myotomy (POEM), and finally surgical myotomy. The choice of therapy should be based on individual characteristics such as gender, patient preference, age, and expertise and comfort with these procedures. Unfortunately, the pathophysiology of achalasia is irreversible, and many of the treatments listed are temporary; therefore, patients require long-term follow-up with the likelihood of repetitive or alternative procedures and treatments [58].

## *Operation*

A laparoscopic Heller myotomy is the gold standard, the most common operative procedure for achalasia treatment [59], and was originally described in 1913 by Ernest Heller. Since that time, the operation itself has been modified several times [60]. Minimally invasive techniques are most commonly performed, with an open procedure available if needed. The esophagus can be approached via the thorax or the abdomen [61, 62]. The surgeon must gain access to the stomach and distal esophagus for dissection. The distal mediastinal esophagus must be mobilized to allow for sufficient length to perform the needed myotomy incision to divide the LES. This ensures a tension-free fundoplication [63].

The myotomy is performed by dividing individual gastric and esophageal muscle fibers in layers, first the longitudinal fibers followed by the circular fibers [2]. When performing the myotomy, a lighted bougie dilator usually 50 Fr or an endoscope may be used to help facilitate muscle dissection and division. When the myotomy is complete, endoscopic inspection is completed to ensure there are no mucosal injuries or issues with the myotomy [63].

Frequently, when performing a Heller myotomy, reflux can occur due to the disruption of the LES; therefore, a Heller myotomy may be combined with an antireflux procedure (described in the GERD section) [11, 64]. When an antireflux procedure is indicated, a partial (Toupet or Dor) versus circumferential (Nissen) wrap is usually completed (described in the GERD section) [65]. A randomized study done including 43 patients who underwent a myotomy for achalasia found that adding a Dor (anterior) fundoplication had significantly fewer GERD symptoms (9% vs. 48%) and lower acid exposure time in the distal esophagus when compared to those who underwent myotomy alone [66].

## *Postoperative Management*

After undergoing minimally invasive Heller myotomy with or without fundoplication, patients are admitted to the hospital after surgery and started on a liquid diet. Patients who underwent a minimally invasive procedure should expect to be discharged in 1–2 days. Depending on surgeon preference, patients may undergo a swallow study (either barium or gastrografin) to assess the integrity of the esophagus and ensure no mucosal injuries. Similar to the postoperative management of GERD, the postoperative management of achalasia is mostly dependent on the symptoms that relate to dysphagia that may occur in the immediate postoperative period. This may be due to inflammation and swelling of the wrap itself. These symptoms usually improve over time; however, if dysphagia becomes an issue, it can be managed with diet modifications and a continued liquid diet. If the dysphagia continues for more than 12 weeks, it requires further work-up. Some patients may require endoscopic dilatation or modification of their wrap [54]. Some patients may still develop postoperative GERD in long-term follow-up; however, it can usually be managed medically (H2 blockers or PPI) [67].

Another concern postoperatively is the recurrence of dysphagia, which can be due to an incomplete myotomy, scar fibrosis and shrinkage, narrowing of the fundoplication [68]. Recurrent dysphagia can be seen in about 3–10% of patients, with symptoms occurring 6 months or later [69]. Other complications that may occur are similar to the postoperative complications described in the GERD section, including gastric or esophageal perforation (1–7%) or pneumothorax [69]. Severe pain, intractable emesis, fever, tachycardia, or leukocytosis should prompt immediate evaluation for a possible perforated viscus.

The advantages of surgical myotomy include initial high success rates and lower rates of symptom recurrence compared to pneumatic dilation [66]. A minimally invasive Heller myotomy is typically associated with a fast recovery and quick return to daily activities, a short hospital stay (1–2 days), and a minimal postoperative pain [2]. Studies have shown that 90–95% of patients continue to have improved symptomatology at 5 years and 80–90% at 10 years [2].

## Conclusion

Benign esophageal disease covers a broad spectrum of pathology including gastrointestinal reflux disease (GERD), hiatal hernia, and achalasia. These disease processes can be managed through a variety of approaches. Medical therapy may often be appropriate initially in managing patients with benign esophageal disease. However, in symptomatic patients, surgery offers an excellent option for definitive therapy in appropriately selected patients. When evaluating patients with benign esophageal disease, it is essential to consider minimally invasive surgical options that may significantly improve and effectively treat their conditions. In such cases, appropriate surgical referrals should be made.

# References

1. Kahrilas PJ, Talley NJ, Grover S. Clinical manifestations and diagnosis of gastroesophageal reflux in adults. In: Basow DS, editor. UpToDate. Waltham: UpToDate; 2008.
2. Fisichella PM, Soper NJ, Pellegrini CA, Patti MG. Surgical management of benign esophageal disorders. London: Springer; 2016.
3. Vakil N, Van Zanten SV, Kahrilas P, Dent J, Jones R. The Montreal definition and classification of gastroesophageal reflux disease: a global evidence-based consensus. Am J Gastroenterol. 2006;101(8):1900.
4. Kamolz T, Pointner R. Laparoscopic refundoplication with prosthetic hiatal closure for recurrent hiatal hernia after primary failed antireflux surgery. Arch Surg. 2003;138(8):902–7.
5. Nebel OT, Fornes MF, Castell DO. Symptomatic gastroesophageal reflux: incidence and precipitating factors. Dig Dis Sci. 1976;21(11):953–6.
6. Barrett NR. Hiatus hernia. A review of some controversial points. Br J Surg. 1954;42(173):231–44.
7. DeVault KR, Castell DO. Updated guidelines for the diagnosis and treatment of gastroesophageal reflux disease. Am J Gastroenterol. 2005;100(1):190.
8. Little AG. Mechanisms of action of antireflux surgery: theory and fact. World J Surg. 1992;16(2):320–5.
9. Landreneau RJ, Del Pino M, Santos R. Management of paraesophageal hernias. Surg Clin North Am. 2005;85(3):411–32.
10. Goyal RK. Chapter 286. Diseases of the esophagus. In: Harrison's principles of internal medicine. 17th ed; 2008.
11. Campos GM, Vittinghoff E, Rabl C, Takata M, Gadenstätter M, Lin F, Ciovica R. Endoscopic and surgical treatments for achalasia: a systematic review and meta-analysis. Ann Surg. 2009;249:45–57.
12. Sadowski DC, Ackah F, Jiang B, Svenson LW. Achalasia: incidence, prevalence and survival. A population-based study. Neurogastroenterol Motil. 2010;22(9):e256–61.
13. Pettit M. Treatment of gastroesophageal reflux disease. Pharm World Sci. 2005;27(6):432–5.
14. Badillo R, Francis D. Diagnosis and treatment of gastroesophageal reflux disease. World J Gastrointest Pharmacol Ther. 2014;5(3):105.
15. Stefanidis D, Hope WW, Kohn GP, Reardon PR, Richardson WS, Fanelli RD. SAGES guidelines committee. Guidelines for surgical treatment of gastroesophageal reflux disease. Surg Endosc. 2010;24(11):2647–69.
16. Duffy JP, Maggard M, Hiyama DT, Atkinson JB. Laparoscopic Nissen fundoplication improves quality of life in patients with atypical symptoms of gastroesophageal reflux. Am Surg. 2003;69(10):833.
17. Gonsalves N, Policarpio-Nicolas M, Zhang Q, Rao MS, Hirano I. Histopathologic variability and endoscopic correlates in adults with eosinophilic esophagitis. Gastrointest Endosc. 2006;64(3):313–9.
18. Fibbe C, Layer P, Keller J, Strate U, Emmermann A, Zornig C. Esophageal motility in reflux disease before and after fundoplication: a prospective, randomized, clinical, and manometric study. Gastroenterology. 2001;121(1):5–14.
19. Yang H, Watson DI, Kelly J, Lally CJ, Myers JC, Jamieson GG. Esophageal manometry and clinical outcome after laparoscopic Nissen fundoplication. J Gastrointest Surg. 2007;11(9):1126–33.
20. Eren S, Gümüş H, Okur A. A rare cause of intestinal obstruction in the adult: Morgagni's hernia. Hernia. 2003;7(2):97–9.
21. Mittal SK, Awad ZT, Tasset M, Filipi CJ, Dickason TJ, Shinno Y, Marsh RE, Tomonaga TJ, Lerner C. The preoperative predictability of the short esophagus in patients with stricture or paraesophageal hernia. Surg Endosc. 2000;14(5):464–8.
22. Morcos SK. Effects of radiographic contrast media on the lung. Br J Radiol. 2003; 76(905):290–5.

23. Eren S, Çiriş F. Diaphragmatic hernia: diagnostic approaches with review of the literature. Eur J Radiol. 2005;54(3):448–59.
24. Swanstrom LL, Jobe BA, Kinzie LR, Horvath KD. Esophageal motility and outcomes following laparoscopic paraesophageal hernia repair and fundoplication. Am J Surg. 1999;177(5):359–63.
25. Vaezi MF, Richter JE. Diagnosis and management of achalasia. Am J Gastroenterol. 1999;94(12):3406–12.
26. Gordon C, Kang JY, Neild PJ, Maxwell JD. The role of the hiatus hernia in gastro-oesophageal reflux disease. Aliment Pharmacol Ther. 2004;20:719–32.
27. Scheffer RC, Bredenoord AJ, Hebbard GS, Smout AJ, Samsom M. Effect of proximal gastric volume on hiatal hernia. Neurogastroenterol Motil. 2010;22:552–6, e120.
28. Stefanidis D, Hope WW, Kohn GP, Reardon PR, Richardson WS, Fanelli RD. Guidelines for surgical treatment of gastroesophageal reflux disease. Surg Endosc. 2010;24:2647–69.
29. Kohn GP, Price RR, Demeester SR, et al. Guidelines for the management of hiatal hernia. Surg Endosc. 2013;27(12):4409–28.
30. Velanovich V, Karmy-Jones R. Surgical management of paraesophageal hernias: outcome and quality of life analysis. Dig Surg. 2001;18:432–7; discussion 437–438.
31. Watson DI, Davies N, Devitt PG, Jamieson GG. Importance of dissection of the hernial sac in laparoscopic surgery for large hiatal hernias. Arch Surg. 1999;134:1069–73.
32. Mattioli S, Lugaresi M, Ruffato A, et al. Collis-Nissen gastroplasty for short oesophagus. Multimed Man Cardiothorac Surg. 2015; https://doi.org/10.1093/mmcts/mmv032.
33. Frantzides CT, Madan AK, Carlson MA, Stavropoulos GP. A prospective, randomized trial of laparoscopic polytetrafluoroethylene (PTFE) patch repair vs simple cruroplasty for large hiatal hernia. Arch Surg. 2002;137:649–52.
34. Granderath FA, Schweiger UM, Kamolz T, Asche KU, Pointner R. Laparoscopic Nissen fundoplication with prosthetic hiatal closure reduces postoperative intrathoracic wrap herniation: preliminary results of a prospective randomized functional and clinical study. Arch Surg. 2005;140:40–8.
35. Oelschlager BK, Pellegrini CA, Hunter J, Soper N, Brunt M, Sheppard B, Jobe B, Polissar N, Mitsumori L, Nelson J, Swanstrom L. Biologic prosthesis reduces recurrence after laparoscopic paraesophageal hernia repair: a multicenter, prospective, randomized trial. Ann Surg. 2006;244:481–90.
36. Morris-Stiff G, Hassn A. Laparoscopic paraoesophageal hernia repair: fundoplication is not usually indicated. Hernia. 2008;12:299–302.
37. Poncet G, Robert M, Roman S, Boulez JC. Laparoscopic repair of large hiatal hernia without prosthetic reinforcement: late results and relevance of anterior gastropexy. J Gastrointest Surg. 2010;14:1910.
38. Rosenberg J, Jacobsen B, Fischer A. Fast-track giant paraesophageal hernia repair using a simplified laparoscopic 23/24 technique. Langenbeck's Arch Surg. 2006;391:38–42.
39. Larusson HJ, Zingg U, Hahnloser D, Delport K, Seifert B, Oertli D. Predictive factors for morbidity and mortality in patients undergoing laparoscopic paraesophageal hernia repair: age, ASA score and operation type influence morbidity. World J Surg. 2009;33(5):980–5.
40. Luketich JD, Nason KS, Christie NA, et al. Outcomes after a decade of laparoscopic giant paraesophageal hernia repair. J Thorac Cardiovasc Surg. 2010;139(2):395–404, 404.e1.
41. Rathore MA, Andrabi SI, Bhatti MI, Najfi SM, Mcmurray A. Metaanalysis of recurrence after laparoscopic repair of paraesophageal hernia. JSLS. 2007;11(4):456–60.
42. Spechler SJ, Goyal RK. The columnar-lined esophagus, intestinal metaplasia, and Norman Barrett. Gastroenterology. 1996;110:614–21.
43. Field SK, Gelfand GA, Mcfadden SD. The effects of antireflux surgery on asthmatics with gastroesophageal reflux. Chest. 1999;116(3):766–74.
44. Prasad GA, Wu TT, Wigle DA, Buttar NS, Wongkeesong LM, Dunagan KT, Lutzke LS, Borkenhagen LS, Wang KK. Endoscopic and surgical treatment of mucosal (T1a) esophageal adenocarcinoma in Barrett's esophagus. Gastroenterology. 2009;137:815–23.

45. Pohl H, Sonnenberg A, Strobel S, Eckardt A, Rosch T. Endoscopic versus surgical therapy for early cancer in Barrett's esophagus: a decision analysis. Gastrointest Endosc. 2009;70:623–34.
46. El-Serag HB. Time trends of gastroesophageal reflux disease: a systematic review. Clin Gastroenterol Hepatol. 2007;5(1):17–26.
47. Engstrom C, Blomqvist A, Dalenback J, Lonroth H, Ruth M, Lundell L. Mechanical consequences of short gastric vessel division at the time of laparoscopic total fundoplication. J Gastrointest Surg. 2004;8:442–7.
48. O'Boyle CJ, Watson DI, Jamieson GG, Myers JC, Game PA, Devitt PG. Division of short gastric vessels at laparoscopic Nissen fundoplication: a prospective double-blind randomized trial with 5-year followup. Ann Surg. 2002;235:165–70.
49. Ludemann R, Watson DI, Jamieson GG, Game PA, Devitt PG. Five-year follow-up of a randomized clinical trial of laparoscopic total versus anterior 180 degrees fundoplication. Br J Surg. 2005;92(2):240–3.
50. Cai W, Watson DI, Lally CJ, Devitt PG, Game PA, Jamieson GG. Ten-year clinical outcome of a prospective randomized clinical trial of laparoscopic Nissen versus anterior 180 (degrees) partial fundoplication. Br J Surg. 2008;95:1501–5.
51. Spence GM, Watson DI, Jamiesion GG, Lally CJ, Devitt PG. Single center prospective randomized trial of laparoscopic Nissen versus anterior 90 degrees fundoplication. J Gastrointest Surg. 2006;10:698–705.
52. Sise A, Friedenberg FK. A comprehensive review of gastroesophageal reflux disease and obesity. Obes Rev. 2008;9:194–203.
53. Parrilla P, Martinez de Haro LF, Ortiz A, Munitiz V, Molina J, Bermejo J, Canteras M. Long-term results of a randomized prospective study comparing medical and surgical treatment of Barrett's esophagus. Ann Surg. 2003;237:291–8.
54. Dominitz JA, Dire CA, Billingsley KG, Todd-stenberg JA. Complications and antireflux medication use after antireflux surgery. Clin Gastroenterol Hepatol. 2006;4(3):299–305.
55. Nguyen NT, Dholakia C, Nguyen XM, Reavis K. Outcomes of minimally invasive esophagectomy without pyloroplasty: analysis of 109 cases. Am Surg. 2010;76(10):1135–8.
56. Rosenthal R, Peterli R, Guenin MO, von Flue M, Ackermann C. Laparoscopic antireflux surgery: long term outcomes and quality of life. J Laparoendosc Adv Surg Tech A. 2006;16:557–61.
57. Dughera L, Chiaverina M, Cacciotella L, Cisarò F. Management of achalasia. Clin Exp Gastroenterol. 2011;4:33.
58. Kahrilas PJ. Treating achalasia; more than just flipping a coin. Gut. 2016;65(5):726–7.
59. Spiess AE, Kahrilas PJ. Treating achalasia: from whalebone to laparoscope. JAMA. 1998;280(7):638–42.
60. Torresan F, Ioannou A, Azzaroli F, Bazzoli F. Treatment of achalasia in the era of high-resolution manometry. Annals Gastroenterol. 2015;28(3):301.
61. Ellis FH Jr, Gibb SP, Crozier RE. Esophagomyotomy for achalasia of the esophagus. Ann Surg. 1980;192(2):157.
62. Pai GP, Ellison RG, Rubin JW, Moore HV. Two decades of experience with modified Heller's myotomy for achalasia. Ann Thorac Surg. 1984;38(3):201–6.
63. Rawlings A, Soper NJ, Oelschlager B, Swanstrom L, Matthews BD, Pellegrini C, Pierce RA, Pryor A, Martin V, Frisella MM, Cassera M. Laparoscopic Dor versus Toupet fundoplication following Heller myotomy for achalasia: results of a multicenter, prospective, randomized-controlled trial. Surg Endosc. 2012;26(1):18–26.
64. West RL, Hirsch DP, Bartelsman JF, De Borst JF, Ferwerda G, Tytgat GN, Boeckxstaens GE. Long term results of pneumatic dilation in achalasia followed for more than 5 years. Am J Gastroenterol. 2002;97(6):1346.
65. Stefanidis D, Richardson W, Farrell T, Kohn GP, Augenstein V, Fanelli RD. Guidelines for the surgical treatment of esophageal achalasia. Society of American Gastrointestinal and Endoscopic Surgeons [serial online] [cited 2015 Feb 15]. Available from: http://www.sages.org/publications/guidelines/guidelines-for-the-surgicaltreatment-of-esophageal-achalasia

66. Richards WO, Torquati A, Holzman MD, Khaitan L, Byrne D, Lutfi R, Sharp KW. Heller myotomy versus Heller myotomy with Dor fundoplication for achalasia: a prospective randomized double-blind clinical trial. Ann Surg. 2004;240(3):405.

67. Cuttitta A, Tancredi A, Andriulli A, De Santo E, Fontana A, Pellegrini F, Scaramuzzi R, Scaramuzzi G. Fundoplication after Heller myotomy: a retrospective comparison between Nissen and Dor. Eurasian J Med. 2011;43(3):133.

68. Iqbal A, Tierney B, Haider M, Salinas VK, Karu A, Turaga KK, Mittal SK, Filipi CJ. Laparoscopic re-operation for failed Heller myotomy. Dis Esophagus. 2006;19(3):193–9.

69. Wright AS, Williams CW, Pellegrini CA, Oelschlager BK. Long-term outcomes confirm the superior efficacy of extended Heller myotomy with Toupet fundoplication for achalasia. Surg Endosc. 2007;21(5):713–8.

# Chapter 4
# Malignant: Esophageal Cancers

Anthony Delliturri, Shintaro Chiba, and Igor Brichkov

## Introduction

According to data from the American Cancer Society, the estimated new cases of esophageal carcinoma in the United States during 2017 was 16,940 for both sexes with a male to female ratio of 3.7:1. In addition, the estimated number of deaths from esophageal carcinoma was 15,690 in both sexes with a male to female ratio of 4.3:1 [1]. Male preponderance can be attributed to lifestyle factors such as obesity, diet low in fruits and vegetables, tobacco, and alcohol. Worldwide, the incidence of new esophageal cancers is 440,000, and new deaths are 442,000 making esophageal cancer ranked ninth and sixth as the most common cancer and most frequent cancer-related cause of death, respectively [2].

Esophageal carcinoma is divided into two histological subtypes with different prevalence globally. Worldwide, esophageal squamous cell carcinoma is the most common histological type particularly in areas of Asia, Africa, and Iran. This is attributed to increased tobacco and alcohol consumption. On the other hand, western nations have a higher incidence of adenocarcinoma, which is attributed to the rising rate of obesity, gastroesophageal reflux disease (GERD), and the lower rate of tobacco use [3].

A. Delliturri · S. Chiba
Department of Surgery, Maimonides Medical Center, Brooklyn, NY, USA
e-mail: adelliturri@maimonidesmed.org

I. Brichkov (✉)
Department of Surgery, Maimonides Medical Center, Albert Einstein College of Medicine, Brooklyn, NY, USA

© Springer Nature Switzerland AG 2019                                                  39
C. Rezac, K. Donohue (eds.), *The Internist's Guide to Minimally Invasive Gastrointestinal Surgery*, Clinical Gastroenterology,
https://doi.org/10.1007/978-3-319-96631-1_4

Prognosis of esophageal cancer has improved over the last five decades in developed countries. In the 1960s, the 5-year survival for esophageal cancer was less than 5%. More recently, 5-year survival has increased to approximately 20% based on data from the Surveillance, Epidemiology, and End Results (SEER) cancer database [4]. This could be attributed to improved screening techniques, earlier diagnosis, and therefore earlier interventions, as well as decreased incidence in risk factors especially tobacco and alcohol use [3]. Prognostic factors are based on tumor stage, histology, and comorbid conditions of the patient.

## Squamous Cell Carcinoma

The most common histologic subtype of esophageal cancer is squamous cell carcinoma with high incidence on the African and Asian continents. The incidence throughout Asia is approximately 90%; however, these numbers have been decreasing in other regions around the world like in Europe and North America [5].

The development of squamous cell carcinoma is initiated by exposure to either caustic or carcinogenic substances such as tobacco smoke and alcohol. Interestingly, it has been noted that tobacco and alcohol work synergistically, further increasing development of squamous cell carcinoma [6]. Smoking cessation programs are an effective way of preventing incidence of squamous cell carcinoma [7]. Other risk factors include consumption of hot beverages, accidental/intentional ingestion of sodium hydroxide/lye, and radiation therapy. Consumption of fruits and vegetables has been found to be protective [8].

## Adenocarcinoma

Adenocarcinoma has become the most prevalent type of esophageal carcinoma in western countries despite the decrease in incidence of squamous cell carcinoma worldwide. One theory for this includes the increasing number of obese and morbidly obese individuals in developed countries. The main risk factors include GERD, obesity, and male sex. On the other hand, like in squamous cell carcinoma, the increased consumption of fruits and vegetables has been shown to be protective. Interestingly, *H. pylori* infection is protective against the development of adenocarcinoma. The increased use of antibiotics in society may have inadvertently caused an increased rate of adenocarcinoma [9].

The development of adenocarcinoma through factors such as chronic gastroesophageal reflux disease has been well characterized through the pathology of Barrett's esophagus. Prolonged gastric acid exposure in the lower esophagus begins the transformation of the squamous epithelium to a columnar type of epithelium similar to that of intestinal mucosa (intestinal metaplasia) known as Barrett's esophaguss. Barrett's esophagus itself is not malignant but has been previously considered a precursor to adenocarcinoma. The incidence of malignant transformation in Barrett's esophagus without dysplasia is much lower than previously thought (<1%), and as a result, no specific therapy is required in these patients other than periodic surveillance endoscopy every 3 years. The mechanism by which dysplasia develops within Barrett's mucosa or which patients will develop dysplasia is unclear. Once low-grade dysplasia develops, it may remain low grade requiring more frequent endoscopic surveillance and biopsy every 3–6 months. Endoscopic ablation of the dysplastic esophageal mucosa may be considered at this point in lieu of frequent endoscopy. Once low-grade dysplasia progresses to high-grade dysplasia, therapy is warranted as up to 40% of high-grade dysplasia bares foci of adenocarcinoma within. High-grade dysplasia may quickly progress to invasive adenocarcinoma, and as such, vigilant endoscopic surveillance, ablation, and/or surgery may be necessary [10].

## Patient Presentation

The clear majority of patients are males who present following a period of dysphagia that begins with difficulty consuming solids followed by liquids [11]. This progression of dysphagia is associated with the tumor burden occluding the lumen of the esophagus. In most cases, this progression is over a period where the patient adapts by consuming smaller bites followed by only liquids. Most patients, who deal with the symptoms over a long period of time, present with involuntary weight loss further adding difficulty to the recovery following surgery to debulk the tumor.

Patients who present with an eventual diagnosis of adenocarcinoma typically report a long period of reflux symptoms [12]. In addition, there has been a link between adenocarcinoma and obesity [13]. The exact pathophysiologic mechanism has yet to be elucidated; however, it could be associated with the patients increased likelihood of developing gastroesophageal reflux disease. Other locally invasive symptoms include hoarseness secondary to invasion of the recurrent laryngeal nerve or pneumonia secondary to tracheoesophageal fistula or chronic aspiration from esophageal obstruction.

## Diagnosis and Staging

Prior to a diagnosis of esophageal cancer, the initial workup for suspicious symptoms of dysphagia in addition to history and physical should include contrast esophagography. Lesions on esophagram suggestive of esophageal cancer include the pathognomonic "apple core" lesion. The "apple core" lesion typically occurs with symmetrical and circumferential growth of the tumor. Most of the time, the esophagram will show an irregular asymmetrical mass [14]. Further investigation requires esophagogastroduodenoscopy to inspect the suspicious lesion and to obtain a tissue diagnosis. During endoscopy, it is important to sample from multiple locations as to avoid missing the diagnosis of esophageal cancer. On endoscopic evaluation, carcinoma could appear as solid tumors, ulcerations, friable masses, or strictures from circumferential growth. Endoscopic evaluation is important to establish histologic tissue type [15]. For patients with Barrett's esophagus, biopsies should be obtained in four quadrants at every 1–2 cm of abnormal mucosa to rule out dysplasia and/or carcinoma. This is particularly important in long-segment Barrett's or nodular dysplasia.

Following confirmation of esophageal cancer on biopsy from endoscopy, the next step is staging of the tumor. Staging is required in order to assess the local or regional extent of disease as well as the presence of distant metastasis. Endoscopic ultrasound is the most sensitive test for local or regional metastasis. Although operator dependent, it can assess for depth of tumor invasion as well as nodal involvement. Staging laparoscopy is rarely necessary for pure esophageal cancers but may be worthwhile in tumors involving the gastroesophageal junction and stomach. A full body positron emission tomography-computed tomography (PET-CT) scan should be performed to rule out distant metastatic disease [16].

Staging is based on the TNM classification system from the Union of International Cancer Control. This staging system evaluates primary tumor pathology, regional lymph nodal spread, and metastases [17]. In the most recent update by the American Joint Committee on Cancer, adenocarcinoma and squamous cell carcinoma are divided into two separate classifications (Table 4.1). In addition, any tumor located within 5 cm of gastroesophageal junction is considered esophageal carcinoma [18]. Briefly, tumors limited to the esophageal mucosa are considered T1a. Tumors penetrating to the submucosa are T1b. Tumors involving the esophageal muscle are T2. Tumors penetrating the periesophageal tissues are T3, and tumors invading neighboring structures are T4. Any nodal metastasis is considered N1 (or N2–N3 based on the number of nodes involved), and any distant metastasis is considered M1 (Table 4.2).

## Treatment Overview

Esophageal carcinoma is treated with either chemotherapy, radiation, surgery, endoscopy or a combination of all of the above. Tumors with distant metastasis are treated with platinum-based chemotherapy with or without radiation. In these cases, radiation therapy is given only as a palliative treatment modality to the primary tumor alone. Early-stage tumors without lymph node involvement or metastatic disease may be treated with primary curative surgical therapy or endoscopic therapy. Preoperative neoadjuvant chemoradiotherapy is indicated for locoregionally advanced tumors, large bulky tumors, tumors with T3 depth of invasion, or any tumors with lymph node involvement. Patients who are poor surgical candidates who have otherwise resectable disease are treated with definitive chemoradiation alone with modest results.

**Table 4.1** American Joint Committee on Cancer (AJCC). TNM classification of carcinoma of the esophagus and esophagogastric junction (7th ed., 2010)

| |
|---|
| *Primary tumor (T)* |
| TX Primary tumor cannot be assessed |
| T0 No evidence of primary tumor |
| Tis High-grade dysplasia[a] |
| T1 Tumor invades lamina propria, muscularis mucosae, or submucosa |
| T1a Tumor invades lamina propria or muscularis mucosae |
| T1b Tumor invades submucosa |
| T2 Tumor invades muscularis propria |
| T3 Tumor invades adventitia |
| T4 Tumor invades adjacent structures |
| T4a Resectable tumor invading pleura, pericardium, or diaphragm |
| T4b Unresectable tumor invading other adjacent structures, such as aorta, vertebral body, trachea, etc. |
| *Regional lymph nodes (N)* |
| NX Regional lymph nodes cannot be assessed |
| N0 No regional lymph node metastasis |
| N1 Metastasis in 1–2 regional lymph nodes |
| N2 Metastasis in 3–6 regional lymph nodes |
| N3 Metastasis in seven or more regional lymph nodes |
| *Distant metastasis (M)* |
| M0 No distant metastasis |
| M1 Distant metastasis |

National Comprehensive Cancer Network. Esophageal cancer (Version 2.2017). https://www.nccn.org/professionals/physician_gls/pdf/esophageal
[a]High-grade dysplasia includes all noninvasive neoplastic epithelia that was formerly called carcinoma in situ, a diagnosis that is no longer used for columnar mucosae anywhere in the gastrointestinal tract

## Endoscopic Treatment

Early esophageal cancer can be treated endoscopically as a primary treatment modality. The 2017 National Comprehensive Cancer Network (NCCN) Guidelines recommend primary treatment of Tis, T1a, and T1b tumors without lymphovascular invasion and Barrett's esophagus with endoscopic mucosal resection (EMR), endoscopic submucosal dissection (ESD), or ablation [19]. EMR involves removal of the involved mucosa and a portion of the submucosa by raising the lesion off of the underlying esophageal muscle by injection and snaring the raised area using an electrosurgical snare. The area that can be removed by this method is limited in size, and larger lesions have to be removed piecemeal. This technique is also limited in terms of ability to assess margins of the resected lesion(s). ESD involves a precise removal of the mucosa and submucosa with margins by using a specialized endoscopic electrosurgical knife through the endoscope. This technique allows for resection of larger superficial esophageal cancers with precise margins. Entire

**Table 4.2** Esophageal cancer staging

*Squamous Cell Carcinoma**

| Stage | T | N | M | Grade | Tumor Location** |
|---|---|---|---|---|---|
| Stage 0 | Tis (HGD) | N0 | M0 | 1, X | Any |
| Stage IA | T1 | N0 | M0 | 1, X | Any |
| Stage IB | T1 | N0 | M0 | 2–3 | Any |
|  | T2–3 | N0 | M0 | 1, X | Lower, X |
| Stage IIA | T2–3 | N0 | M0 | 1, X | Upper, middle |
|  | T2–3 | N0 | M0 | 2–3 | Lower, X |
| Stage IIB | T2–3 | N0 | M0 | 2–3 | Upper, middle |
|  | T1–2 | N1 | M0 | Any | Any |
| Stage IIIA | T1–2 | N2 | M0 | Any | Any |
|  | T3 | N1 | M0 | Any | Any |
|  | T4a | N0 | M0 | Any | Any |
| Stage IIIB | T3 | N2 | M0 | Any | Any |
| Stage IIIC | T4a | N1–2 | M0 | Any | Any |
|  | T4b | Any | M0 | Any | Any |
|  | Any | N3 | M0 | Any | Any |
| Stage IV | Any | Any | M1 | Any | Any |

*Or mixed histology including a squamous component or NOS.

**Location of the primary cancer site is defined by the position of the upper (proximal) edge of the tumor in the esophagus.

*Adenocarcinoma*

| Stage | T | N | M | Grade |
|---|---|---|---|---|
| Stage 0 | Tis (HGD) | N0 | M0 | 1, X |
| Stage IA | T1 | N0 | M0 | 1-2, X |
| Stage IB | T1 | N0 | M0 | 3 |
|  | T2 | N0 | M0 | 1-2, X |
| Stage IIA | T2 | N0 | M0 | 3 |
| Stage IIB | T3 | N0 | M0 | Any |
|  | T1–2 | N1 | M0 | Any |
| Stage IIIA | T1–2 | N2 | M0 | Any |
|  | T3 | N1 | M0 | Any |
|  | T4a | N0 | M0 | Any |
| Stage IIIB | T3 | N2 | M0 | Any |
| Stage IIIC | T4a | N1–2 | M0 | Any |
|  | T4b | Any | M0 | Any |
|  | Any | N3 | M0 | Any |
| Stage IV | Any | Any | M1 | Any |

**Histologic Grade (G)**

GX  Grade cannot be assessed – stage grouping as G1
G1  Well differentiated
G2  Moderately differentiated
G3  Poorly differentiated
G4  Undifferentiated - stage grouping as G3 squamous

National Comprehensive Cancer Network. Esophageal cancer (Version 2.2017). https://www.nccn.org/professionals/physician_gls/pdf/esophageal

circumferential lesions may be resected with this technique. The limitations of the technique include a higher perforation risk, significantly longer procedure time, and limited number of endoscopists who are comfortable with this procedure.

Ablation of the esophageal mucosa may be accomplished using a radiofrequency (RFA) energy device introduced endoscopically which ablates mucosa to a depth of 1 mm. Typically, a total of two treatments to a given site are performed at each treatment session with 2–3 treatments required to successfully ablate all affected mucosa. With this technique, large portions of the esophageal mucosa may be ablated, and it is the only modality that has shown to reverse intestinal metaplasia. Originally developed for the ablation of Barrett's esophagus without dysplasia, RFA has been used for Barrett's esophagus with low-grade dysplasia, high-grade dysplasia, as well as invasive carcinoma with success. Due to recent evidence of low risk of malignant transformation in nondysplastic Barrett's esophagus, RFA for these patients is no longer necessary or indicated.

In a large study, 96.3% complete remission was achieved with 0.2% tumor-related death due to metastasis for early-stage mucosal adenocarcinoma [20]. After endoscopic treatment, close surveillance of these patients is necessary with possible repeat endoscopic treatment or surgery due to failure. Complications after endoscopic treatment include bleeding, perforation, and stricture formation.

## Surgical Treatment

Esophagectomy is the primary therapy for early-stage esophageal cancer T2 N0 or T1 tumors amenable to surgical resection [21]. For locoregionally advanced disease, esophagectomy is performed after neoadjuvant chemoradiation in order to achieve complete resection. Occasionally, esophagectomy is performed as a salvage modality for those patients who fail primary definitive chemoradiation.

Surgical options for esophageal cancer include traditional open or minimally invasive approaches. Whether open or minimally invasive, there are several steps of esophagectomy common to both. The principles of surgical resection of esophageal cancer are resection of a portion of the esophagus as well as a portion of the upper stomach. Typically, 10 cm of esophagus proximal to the tumor must be resected as well as 3–4 cm distal. This is due to the likelihood of tumor spread within the extensive lymphatic drainage system within the esophageal submucosa. Due to the anatomic fixation of the esophagus within the thorax, segmental resection of the esophagus with anastomosis is not possible, and esophageal replacement with another tubular structure is necessary. The most commonly used structure is tubularized stomach. In the abdomen, the stomach must be mobilized, and a new esophageal replacement conduit must be fashioned by forming a limited diameter gastric tube. Although the non tubularized stomach has been used, the bulk of a large stomach within the mediastinum may lead to postoperative dysphagia and cardiopulmonary compression. The choice of conduit is primarily the stomach, but if the stomach is not available as a conduit due to prior gastrectomy, the colon or jejunum can be used as an alternative. After mobilizing the stomach and creating the gastric conduit, the esophagus must be mobilized through the hiatus from the abdominal incision or by thoracotomy/thoracoscopy. After the esophagus has been fully mobilized, the esophagus is resected, and the esophagogastrostomy is made in the thoracic cavity or in the neck. The amount of esophagus resected and the location of the anastomosis depend largely on the location of the tumor and also on preoperative radiation and surgeon preference. For tumors of the mid- and upper thoracic esophagus, a near-total esophagectomy needs to be performed in order to obtain negative proximal margins. For lower esophageal or gastro-esophageal junction tumors, a smaller portion of the esophagus requires resection, and the anastomosis can be created in the thorax or in the neck based on surgeon preference. Also, a wide preoperative radiation field may require resection of a longer segment of the esophagus and mandate a cervical anastomosis rather than an intrathoracic one as radiation effects may complicate anastomotic healing.

There are three approaches to perform an esophagectomy which include transhiatal, Ivor Lewis, and McKeown. In the transhiatal or two-field approach, the incision is made in the abdomen and the neck. The distal esophagus is mobilized from the abdomen, and the proximal esophagus is mobilized through a cervical incision with the esophagogastrostomy performed in the neck. No incisions in the thorax are required in this approach as the esophagus is bluntly separated from its intrathoracic attachments by a hand inserted in a paraesophageal manner via the neck incision as well as via the hiatus through an upper midline abdominal incision. As this procedure is performed blindly, a surgeon experienced in esophagectomy is required. This technique may also be performed via a minimally invasive approach (i.e., laparoscopy through the hiatus and manual blunt dissection or video-assisted dissection through the neck incision) (Fig. 4.1). Limitations of this approach include difficulty in dissection of certain bulky tumors and bleeding from blind dissection and limited ability to assess, sample, and resect lymph nodes within the mediastinum. Advantages of this approach include decreased postoperative pulmonary complications and pain from thoracotomy or thoracoscopy. Also for non-bulky tumors located in the distal esophagus or GEJ that are amenable to a laparoscopic transhiatal esophagectomy, this approach allows for earlier postoperative recovery less pain with equivalent rates of complete surgical resection and cure.

The Ivor Lewis esophagogastrectomy is also a two-field (or two-incision) approach. The stomach is mobilized from the abdomen, and the distal and the mid-thoracic esophagus is dissected via right thoracotomy/thoracoscopy and esophago-gastrostomy performed in the chest. The advantage of this approach is that the mediastinal lymph nodes can be dissected under direct vision unlike in the transhiatal approach where most of the esophageal dissection is performed blindly through the abdomen. For distal esophageal cancer where it is unnecessary to resect any of the proximal esophagus, the Ivor Lewis approach is appropriate. Experienced surgeons will perform this technique via a minimally invasive approach [laparoscopy for the abdominal portion and thoracoscopy for the intrathoracic portion (Fig. 4.2)]. Disadvantages of this technique include added pain and associated pulmonary complications from thoracic incisions as well as risk of significant morbidity associated with a potential intrathoracic anastomotic complication. However, using minimally invasive techniques, the pulmonary and pain complications associated with thora-

**Fig. 4.1** Incisions
performed for a
minimally invasive
transhiatal
esophagectomy

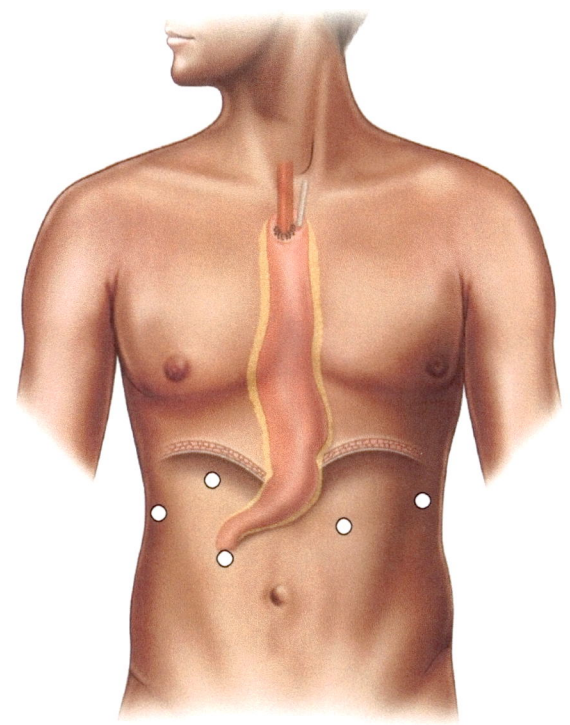

cotomy are limited. The benefits of the Ivor Lewis technique include direct visualization during dissection of the intrathoracic esophagus and better access to mediastinal
lymph nodes. Compared to other approaches, there is no proven oncologic-related
approach to one technique over any other technique, but recent retrospective data
shows increased number of lymph nodes obtained with minimally invasive esophagectomy compared to open without any difference in morbidity and mortality [22].

A third less common approach to esophagectomy is the three-field (or three-
incision) approach named after McKeown. The McKeown technique combines the
techniques, advantages, and disadvantages of both transhiatal and Ivor Lewis
approaches. The surgeon starts the operation with the dissection of the thoracic esophagus via right thoracotomy allowing for direct visual access to both the esophagus and
mediastinal lymph nodes. Then the patient is laid supine, and cervical and abdominal
incisions are made as for a transhiatal esophagectomy (Fig. 4.3). The stomach is mobilized in the abdomen and proximal esophagus dissected through the cervical incision.
The conduit is passed through the chest blindly, and esophagogastrostomy is performed in the neck. The potential benefit of having a cervical anastomosis is decreased
morbidity of anastomotic leak in the neck and increased length of proximal esophagus
resected with the added benefit of extensive intrathoracic lymphadenectomy.
Additionally, direct visual access to the intrathoracic esophagus limits potential injuries to intrathoracic structures associated with blind dissection as in the transhiatal

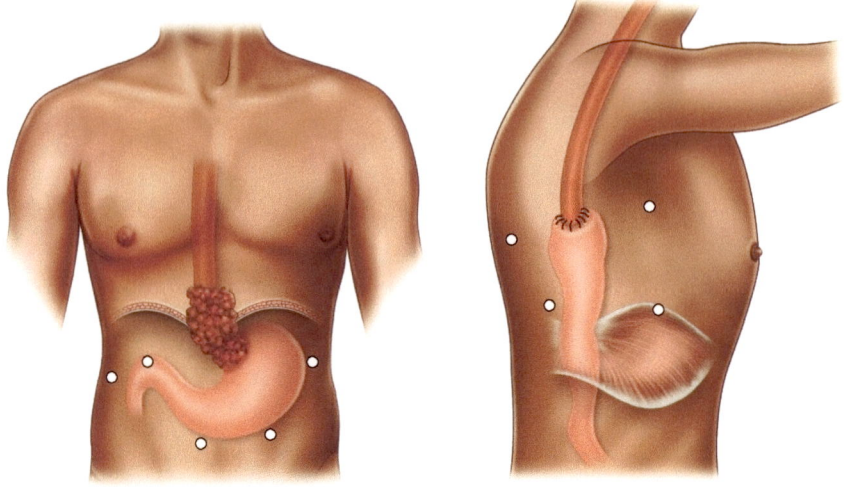

**Fig. 4.2** Incisions performed for a minimally invasive Ivor Lewis esophagectomy

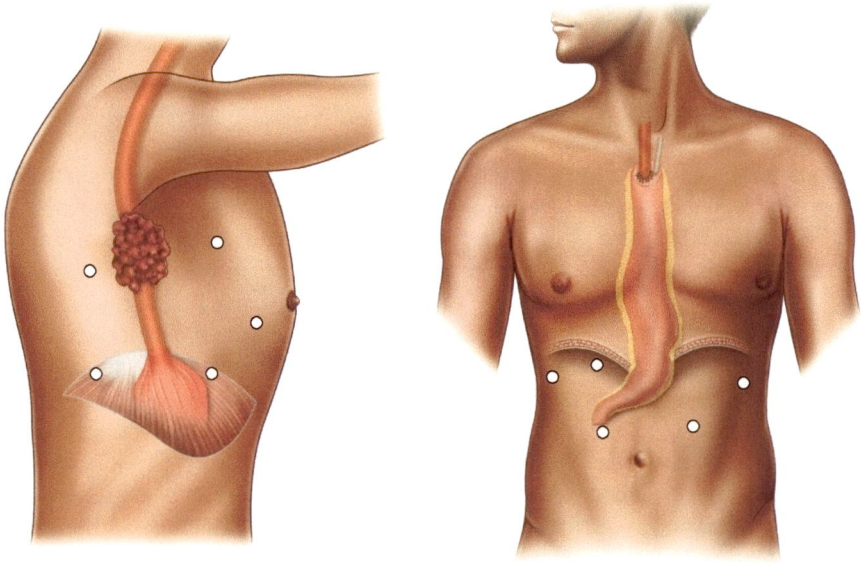

**Fig. 4.3** Incisions performed for a minimally invasive McKeown esophagectomy

approach. The largest disadvantage of this technique is increased pain and pulmonary complication associated with thoracic incisions though this is limited if thoracic esophageal mobilization is performed thoracoscopically. Mid-esophageal bulky tumors with suspected lymph node involvement or mid-esophageal tumors treated with neoadjuvant intrathoracic radiation are best treated via the McKeown technique.

Open surgical approaches which include both laparotomy and thoracotomy incisions result in significant postoperative morbidity. Comparing open and minimally invasive techniques, there was a reduction in hospital stay and total number of complications with laparoscopy [22–24]. A recent meta-analysis shows that overall complication rates were lower in the minimally invasive group, specifically pulmonary complications, wound infection rates, and intraoperative blood loss, but no difference in overall long-term survival [22, 25]. The lower complication rate for minimally invasive approach may be secondary to unopened abdomen and chest. In recent years, robotic-assisted esophagectomy has also been performed with equivalent short-term oncologic outcomes, no increased morbidity, and equivalent numbers of lymph nodes harvested [22]. Further investigation should be performed for this novel approach, and a randomized controlled trial is underway to further investigate the utility of robotics for esophagectomy [26].

Preoperatively, risks, benefits, and postoperative expectations should be discussed with the patient and caregivers. On the day of surgery, the patient should be nil per os overnight per anesthesia protocol at an individual institution. To control the pain postoperatively, possible epidural placement should be discussed with the anesthesia team if a thoracotomy is anticipated.

Postoperatively, the patient may require ventilator support depending on the length of the operation, intraoperative complication/difficulty, presence of a thoracotomy incision, and surgeon preference. Surgical intensive care is frequently appropriate for monitoring of the patients immediately perioperatively as patients require monitoring for pulmonary complication, bleeding, and arrhythmias. A nasogastric tube is routinely placed through esophagogastrostomy anastomosis to keep the gastric conduit decompressed until the anastomosis is given the time to heal. Anastomosis in the neck or thorax depending on surgical technique used may be drained via a closed suction drain which is removed after anastomotic healing has taken place. We routinely perform an esophagram on postoperatively day 5 to rule out an anastomotic leak before taking out the nasogastric tube and starting a liquid diet.

If a thoracotomy/thoracoscopy is performed, a chest drain is left in place to drain the anastomosis in case of an anastomotic leak if the esophagogastrostomy is in the chest, as well as to allow for reexpansion of the lung and drainage of any pleural effusions. Prophylactic antibiotics would be given perioperatively, but it is not necessary to continue the antibiotics postoperatively unless complicated by anastomotic leak, mediastinitis, surgical site infection, or pneumonia. Deep vein thrombosis prophylaxis with low-molecular-weight heparin and sequential compression stocking should be given perioperatively to decrease incidence of deep vein thrombosis and subsequent pulmonary emboli [27].

# Outcomes

Complications after esophagectomy include anastomotic leak, wound infection, pulmonary complication, recurrent laryngeal nerve injury, anastomotic stricture, arrhythmia, pulmonary emboli, deep vein thrombosis, and postoperative bleeding. Complication specific to esophagectomy will be discussed in detail.

Anastomotic leaks can present as pain, tenderness, fever, tachycardia, and leukocytosis. Esophagram or computed tomography (CT) scan with oral contrast is diagnostic. Comparing cervical and intrathoracic anastomotic leaks, the former is considered to be less morbid. An anastomotic leak can be treated nonoperatively if it is contained or drained by closed suction drain or a chest tube. If there is no proper drainage, the leak must be controlled by image-guided drain placement or reoperation. Endoscopic therapies for anastomotic leaks include clipping and stenting for patients that are not septic and hemodynamically stable. Depending on the institution, these interventions are performed by gastroenterologists or thoracic/general surgeons. More novel approach is an endoluminal drainage of the leak with a vacuum-assisted closure system, but there is very limited data for this approach, and it is currently under further investigation.

Anastomotic stricture is a late complication for an esophagectomy. Patient may complain of dysphagia, food intolerance, nausea, vomiting, and chest pain. An esophagram is the initial diagnostic tool, and it should be followed by endoscopy. Endoscopic dilation with bougienage or balloon is the primary mode of therapy for esophageal strictures [28]. Various injections of steroids have been attempted with varying benefits. Repeat dilations may be necessary for resolution of the symptoms.

Recurrent laryngeal nerve (RLN) injury occurs in approximately 1% of the population after esophagectomy [29], particularly when dissection in the neck was used. RLN innervates all intrinsic muscles of the larynx except for the cricothyroid, and damage to the nerve causes changes in voice, phonation, swallowing, and coughing. Fiberoptic endoscopy is diagnostic for RLN injury. If there is an injury, an intervention is usually deferred for 6 months to a year as there is the potential for RLN to regain function by nerve regeneration. Vocal cord injection is usually the first-line therapy. If the symptoms do not improve and are refractory to the injections, laryngoplasty, arytenoid adduction, and cricothyroid subluxation are procedures to medialize the cord anatomically.

# Summary and Conclusion

Esophageal cancer continues to be associated with significant mortality worldwide. Esophageal carcinoma can be squamous cell carcinoma or adenocarcinoma, the latter increasing in frequency is North America and Europe. Obesity and reflux disease have been attributed to the cause.

Patients with esophageal cancer frequently present with dysphagia and weight loss. Once suspected, esophagography and endoscopy are diagnostic. Esophageal cancers are staged using endoscopic ultrasonography and computed tomography to assess for depth of invasion, nodal disease, and distant metastatic disease.

Early-stage esophageal cancers can be treated endoscopically avoiding the need for other modalities, while locoregionally advanced tumors require chemotherapy with radiation followed by surgery. Surgery requires esophagectomy and partial gastrectomy with replacement of the resected esophagus with a suitable tubularized replacement conduit, most commonly the stomach. Three methods of performing esophagectomy are described including the transhiatal, Ivor Lewis, and McKeown. Each technique has specific advantages and disadvantages, but preference for either technique is largely based on surgeon preference. All techniques can be safely performed in a minimally invasive fashion by experienced surgeons.

# References

1. Siegel RL, Miller KD, Jemal A. Cancer statistics, 2017. CA Cancer J Clin. 2017;67:7–30.
2. Global Burden of Disease Cancer Collaboration. The global burden of cancer 2013. JAMA Oncol. 2015;1(4):505–27.
3. Zhang H-Z, Jin G-F, Shen H-B. Epidemiologic differences in esophageal cancer between Asian and Western populations. Chin J Cancer. 2012;31(6):281–6.
4. Njei B, McCarty TR, Birk JW. Trends in esophageal cancer survival in United States adults from 1973 to 2009: a SEER database analysis. J Gastroenterol Hepatol. 2016;31(6):1141–6.
5. Arnold M, Soerjomataram I, Ferlay J, Forman D. Global incidence of oesophageal cancer by histological subtype in 2012. Gut. 2015;64:381–7.
6. Prabhu A, Obi KO, Rubenstein JH. The synergistic e ects of alcohol and tobacco consumption on the risk of esophageal squamous cell carcinoma: a meta-analysis. Am J Gastroenterol. 2014;109:822–7.
7. Bosetti C, Gallus S, Garavello W, La Vecchia C. Smoking cessation and the risk of oesophageal cancer: an overview of published studies. Oral Oncol. 2006;42:957–64.
8. Liu J, Wang J, Leng Y, Lv C. Intake of fruit and vegetables and risk of esophageal squamous cell carcinoma: A meta-analysis of observational studies. Int J Cancer. 2013;133:473–85.
9. Lagergren J, Lagergren P. Recent developments in esophageal adenocarcinoma. CA Cancer J Clin. 2013;63:232–48.
10. Spechler SJ, Souza RF. Barrett's esophagus. N Engl J Med. 2014;371:836–45.
11. Gibbs JF, Rajput A, Chadha KS, et al. The changing profile of esophageal cancer presentation and its implication for diagnosis. J Natl Med Assoc. 2007;99(6):620–6.
12. Chai J, Jamal MM. Esophageal malignancy: A growing concern. World J Gastroenterol. 2012;18(45):6521–6.
13. Arnold M, Colquhoun A, Cook MB, Ferlay J, Forman D, Soerjomataram I. Obesity and the incidence of upper gastrointestinal cancers: an ecological approach to examine differences across age and sex. Cancer Epidemiol Biomarkers Prev. 2016;25(1):90–7.
14. Levine MS, Chu P, Furth EE, Rubesin SE, Laufer I, Herlinger H. Carcinoma of the esophagus and esophagogastric junction: sensitivity of radiographic diagnosis. AJR Am J Roentgenol. 1997;168:1423–6.
15. Rice TW, Blackstone EH, Rusch VW. A cancer staging primer: esophagus and esophagogastric junction. J Thorac Cardiovasc Surg. 2010;139:527–9.

16. Desai RK, Tagliabue JR, Wegryn SA, Einstein DM. CT evaluation of wall thickening in the alimentary tract. Radiographics. 1991;11:771–83.
17. Brierley JD, Gospodarowicz MK, Wittekind C. TNM classification of malignant tumours. 8th ed. Hoboken: Wiley-Blackwell; 2016.
18. Amin MB, Greene FL, Edge SB, Compton CC, Gershenwald JE, Brookland RK, Meyer L, Gress DM, Byrd DR, Winchester DP. The Eighth Edition AJCC Cancer Staging Manual: Continuing to build a bridge from a population-based to a more "personalized" approach to cancer staging. CA Cancer J Clin. 2017;67:93–9.
19. National Comprehensive Cancer Network. Esophageal cancer (Version 2.2017). https://www.nccn.org/professionals/physician_gls/pdf/esophageal
20. Pech O, May A, Manner H, Behrens A, Pohl J, Weferling M, Hartmann U, Manner N, Huijsmans J, Gossner L, Rabenstein T, Vieth M, Stolte M, Ell C. Long-term efficacy and safety of endoscopic resection for patients with mucosal adenocarcinoma of the esophagus. Gastroenterology. 2014;146(3):652–660.e1.
21. Mariette C, Dahan L, Mornex F, et al. Surgery alone versus chemoradiotherapy followed by surgery for stage I and II esophageal cancer: nal analysis of randomized controlled phase III trial FFCD 9901. J Clin Oncol. 2014;32:2416–22.
22. Yerokun BA, Sun Z, Yang CJ, Gulack BC, Speicher PJ, Adam MA, D'Amico TA, Onaitis MW, Harpole DH, Berry MF, Hartwig MG. Minimally invasive versus open esophagectomy for esophageal cancer: a population-based analysis. Ann Thorac Surg. 2016;102(2):416–23. https://doi.org/10.1016/j.athoracsur.2016.02.078. Epub 2016 May 4.
23. Gurusamy KS, Pallari E, Midya S, Mughal M. Laparoscopic versus opentranshiatal oesophagectomy for oesophageal cancer. Cochrane Database Syst Rev. 2016;3:CD011390.
24. Yibulayin W, Abulizi S, Lv H, Sun W. Minimally invasive oesophagectomy versus open esophagectomy for resectable esophageal cancer: a meta-analysis. World J Surg Oncol. 2016;14(1):304.
25. Guo W, Ma X, Yang S, Zhu X, Qin W, Xiang J, Lerut T, Li H. Combined thoracoscopic-laparoscopic esophagectomy versus open esophagectomy: ameta-analysis of outcomes. Surg Endosc. 2016;30(9):3873–81. https://doi.org/10.1007/s00464-015-4692-x. Epub 2015 Dec 10.
26. van der Sluis PC, Ruurda JP, van der Horst S, Verhage RJ, Besselink MG, Prins MJ, Haverkamp L, Schippers C, Rinkes IH, Joore HC, Ten Kate FJ, Koffijberg H, Kroese CC, van Leeuwen MS, Lolkema MP, Reerink O, Schipper ME, Steenhagen E, Vleggaar FP, Voest EE, Siersema PD, van Hillegersberg R. Robot-assisted minimally invasive thoraco-laparoscopic esophagectomy versus open transthoracic esophagectomy for resectable esophageal cancer, a randomized controlled trial (ROBOT trial). Trials. 2012;13:230.
27. Farge D, Bounameaux H, Brenner B, Cajfinger F, Debourdeau P, Khorana AA, Pabinger I, Solymoss S, Douketis J, Kakkar A. International clinical practice guidelines including guidance for direct oral anticoagulants in the treatment and prophylaxis of venous thromboembolism in patients with cancer. Lancet Oncol. 2016;17(10):e452–66.
28. Raymondi R, Pereira-Lima JC, Valves A, Morales GF, Marques D, Lopes CV, Marroni CA. Endoscopic dilation of benign esophageal strictures without fluoroscopy: experience of 2750 procedures. Hepato-Gastroenterology. 2008;55(85):1342–8.
29. Luketich JD, Pennathur A, Awais O, Levy RM, Keeley S, Shende M, Christie NA, Weksler B, Landreneau RJ, Abbas G, Schuchert MJ, Nason KS. Outcomes after minimally invasive esophagectomy: review of over 1000 patients. Ann Surg. 2012;256(1):95–103.

# Chapter 5
# Esophageal Surgery

**Navid Ajabshir, Daniela Treitl, Anthony Andreoni, and Kfir Ben-David**

## Introduction

Spanning from the neck to the stomach, the esophagus is often intuitively considered a simple structure. It isn't until pathology strikes; however, that its complexity is revealed. Surgical care involving this dynamic, tube-like vacuum may be wrought with complication without sufficient understanding and careful planning. Unfortunately, the relative paucity of global pathology precludes the medical community from having a robust, widespread knowledge of treatment modalities available to patients. This may translate to a potential relative uncertainty when an out-of-scope provider counsels their patients.

## Motility Disorders

The musculature of the esophagus involves an outer thick longitudinal muscle with an inner circular layer. The upper 6 cm of the esophagus contains striated muscle, and the lower two thirds containing involuntary, smooth muscles. Most clinically important disorders of motility involve the lower part of the esophagus. Patients with motility disorders may present with symptoms such as chest pain, dysphagia, reflux or regurgitation, dysphagia, and weight loss. Of course, these

N. Ajabshir · D. Treitl · K. Ben-David (✉)
Department of Surgery, Mount Sinai Medical Center, Miami Beach, FL, USA
e-mail: Navid.ajabshir@msmc.com; kfir.bendavid@msmc.com

A. Andreoni
Rutgers Robert Wood Johnson Medical School, New Brunswick, NJ, USA

© Springer Nature Switzerland AG 2019                                    53
C. Rezac, K. Donohue (eds.), *The Internist's Guide to Minimally Invasive Gastrointestinal Surgery*, Clinical Gastroenterology,
https://doi.org/10.1007/978-3-319-96631-1_5

are not exclusive to esophageal pathology, and a high clinical acumen must be employed to tease this out. High-resolution manometry with esophageal pressure topography has allowed for a greater level diagnostic detail than what was previously achieved via conventional manometry. Aberrancy in motility may be evident at any point throughout the esophageal tract. It is helpful to categorize such disorders based on the cause, which can be further subdivided into primary versus secondary, and location.

The most salient and well-known example of a primary motility disorder of the esophagus is achalasia, an entity which affects the entirety of the esophagus. Several types exist all of which revolve around the findings that one or more parts of the esophagus "fails to relax." The etiology has yet to be elucidated, although theories are based on a neurogenic degeneration. Patients present with a classic triad of dysphagia which progresses from liquids to solids, regurgitation, and weight loss. The gold standard for diagnosis is manometry; however, a barium swallow esophagram will demonstrate the classic "bird's beak" sign, and a motility study will fail to show a peristaltic wave. As the disease progresses, the esophagus becomes dilated and tortuous, even described as sigmoidal, propagating the dysmotility and lack of coordinated peristalsis. On manometry, there are five pathognomonic findings:

1. Hypertensive lower esophageal sphincter (LES) (>35 mmHg).
2. LES fails to relax with deglutition.
3. Pressure of the body of the esophagus above baseline.
4. Mirrored contractions without peristalsis.
5. Atonic or low-amplitude wave form.

Intervention is aimed toward palliation because while there exist ways to decrease muscular tone, rectifying the motility dysfunction in the body of the esophagus is not possible at this time. Despite severity of symptomatology, patients are encouraged to seek treatment, or at least some form of surveillance, as there is an increased risk of cancer if unchecked [1]. A similar entity known as ineffective esophageal motility (IEM) also affects both the body of the esophagus and the LES. It is diagnosed when greater than 30% of wet swallows are determined to be ineffective on manometry. This entity was first described in 1997 and is often associated with gastroesophageal reflux disease (GERD) [2].

Hypertensive lower esophageal sphincter may present similar to achalasia; however, there is effective peristalsis in the body of the esophagus, whereas with achalasia this is lacking. This entity was first described in the 1960s by Code et al. and is now diagnosed with manometric findings of a median relaxing pressure greater than 15 mmHg, according to the Chicago classification [3]. Treatment is similar to that of achalasia, though may be more definitive.

Diffuse esophageal spasm (DES) involves mainly the body of the esophagus. It is more commonly found in women and often presents as chest pain or dysphagia in the patient with multiple other complaints or at times of increased stress and anxiety. Patients should be asked whether they are experiencing regurgitation of food products or if symptoms worsen with cold fluids. Directed workup may include an outpatient upper gastrointestinal radiograph series to visualize the classic "corkscrew" esophagus or distal "bird's beak" narrowing. Manometric findings include high amplitude (>120 mmHg) or long duration (>2.5 s); however, the spontaneity associated with this condition may render manometry inconclusive. Currently, DES is more likely treated nonsurgically such as with medication (e.g., nitrates, calcium channel blockade, anticholinergic agents) or with endoscopy (e.g., pneumatic balloon dilation, botulinum toxin injection). Intractability or evidence of pulsion diverticula warrants surgical intervention with an esophagomyotomy, described later in the chapter.

Nutcracker, or Jackhammer esophagus, is due to hypertrophic musculature throughout the esophagus. The intense peristaltic waves are of high amplitude. The disease can occur at any age, and patients will present similar to how they would with DES except there is a lack of regurgitation. It is important to keep this in mind, as management is typically nonsurgical. Interestingly, the LES is normal in tone and generally relaxes with wet swallows.

Secondary motility disorders result from patient's having systemic diseases such as collagen, vascular, or neuromuscular disorders. Examples include, but are not limited to, myasthenia gravis, lupus erythematosus, scleroderma, dermatomyositis or polymyositis, and Chagas disease.

Manometry is paramount to the diagnosis and treatment of motility disorders. This first came about in the 1970s and is still widely used today to hone in on functional disorders manifested as dysphagia or odynophagia. Quantifying pressures at different times and locations along the esophagus allows for a more objective diagnosis. Typically, a long, narrow esophageal manometry catheter is passed via the nares to beyond the gastroesophageal junction. There exist a variety of catheters with pressure transducers in multiple configurations. At minimum, these are spaced 5 cm apart and may be radially oriented. With the advent of high-resolution manometry, catheters with 36 transducers can be used to generate spatiotemporal video tracings.

The pressure, abdominal esophagus length, and sphincter length can be determined by passing the catheter tip beyond the LES resting pressure (high) to the respiratory inversion point (low and varies with respiration) and withdrawing back to above the LES (drop in pressure). This pull-through technique may also be used to assess the upper cricopharyngeal sphincter. Further maneuvers include assessment of LES relaxation as well as function of the esophageal body by recording pressure measurements during ten wet swallows (5 mL of water) and correlating these with timing.

Surgical intervention for primary motility disorders typically relies on decreasing hypertonicity. Surgical myotomy (Heller) is pursued when conservative measures (i.e., as nitrates, calcium channel blockers, pneumatic dilation, and botulinum toxin injections) have failed. A Heller myotomy consists of a single incision through the muscle fibers of the GE junction extending from 3 to 4 cm on the stomach to at least 6 cm on the esophagus or as cephalad as possible. This is routinely approached laparoscopically (LHM) with an example of port configuration in Fig. 5.1. In pathology, which traverses a greater span of esophagus than the LES, approach can be through a left video-assisted thoracoscopic surgery. Often, an accompanying partial fundoplication procedure is employed to prevent expectant acid reflux following incision of fibers which include those of the lower esophageal sphincter. Myotomy

**Fig. 5.1** Port configuration
for laparoscopic Heller
myotomy

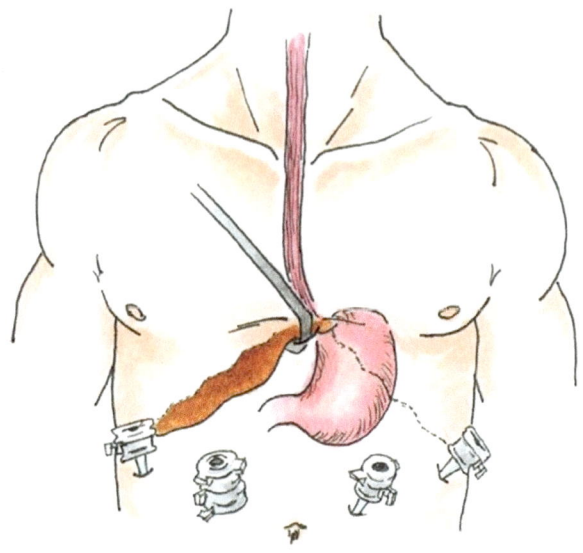

may also be completed endoscopically, known as per-oral endoscopic myotomy (POEM) with good long-term success rates [4]. A meta-analysis including 74 studies and 7700 patients showed higher rates of symptom (dysphagia) relief at 12 and 24 months with POEM compared to laparoscopic Heller myotomy, yet with significantly greater rates of clinical and pathological reflux. On average, patients were hospitalized 1 day greater with LHM [5].

Preoperatively, to reduce undigested food in the esophagus, patients can be on a liquid diet for several days. Recovery from a Heller myotomy is fairly straightforward. Patients should experience immediate relief of symptoms and are safe to resume diet, starting with liquids and advancing to solids. Complications include inadequacy, i.e., failing to fully transect the hypertrophied muscle which may be seen in less than 10% of patients and the dreaded complication of perforation [5]. In the case of the former, repeat surgery or POEM may be necessary. If the latter is discovered, closure and contralateral myotomy may be required.

## Diverticular Disorders

Unchecked motility disorders of the upper esophageal sphincter (UES), lower esophageal sphincter, or esophageal body can lead the formation of diverticula. With dysmotility, elevated pressures lead to herniation of the mucosa and submucosa layers through the muscular layers of the esophagus. Classification can be based on the location such as epiphrenic (supradiaphragmantic), parabronchial (mid-esophageal), and the most commonly thought pharyngoesophageal (Zenker). Pulsion diverticula can occur anywhere throughout the esophagus and are also considered false diverticula. True diverticula with outpouchings of the muscular layer tend to result from inflammatory carinal lymph nodes which contract during healing, although they may result from motility disorders as well.

A Zenker's diverticulum may be asymptomatic initially, then cause a sticking sensation, cough, excess salivation, and subsequently lead to regurgitation of foul-smelling undigested food particles as it progresses. Barium esophagram will readily identify the diverticulum. As this occurs most commonly in the seventh decade of life, complications such as pneumonia or lung abscess can be fatal, and surgical or endoscopic treatment is warranted. Most mid and distal diverticula are asymptomatic and are found incidentally. They are usually on the right side of the esophagus as there exist a greater number of surrounding structures on the left. When identified, it is important to not only characterize with imaging i.e., esophagram or CT but to also diagnose a causal motility disorder with manometry which will also guide treatment. A diverticulum within 10 cm of the gastroesophageal junction is considered an epiphrenic, and endoscopy should be considered to evaluate for mucosal lesions.

Barium swallow radiography can assess both anatomy and motility of the esophagus, though the focus here is to detect structural problems. Patients are typically upright to assess swallow mechanics, supine when assessing for esophageal peristalsis pattern, and prone when evaluating the extent of a hiatal hernia. Filling defects reflect a mass or stricture, whereas pooling or spillage demonstrates a diverticulum or leak, respectively. Barium may be mixed with solid foods such as bread or marshmallows to detect dysphagia that may not occur with liquids. Unfortunately, if relying only on this assessment modality, small neoplasms, mild esophagitis, and varices may be missed. Video or cineradiography is essential to evaluate the fine mechanics of the pharyngeal phase of swallowing.

Diverticular disease can be treated with open surgery or endoscopically. For diverticula <3 cm, the open technique provides greater symptomatic relief [6]. With open surgery, an incision is made through the left side of the neck, anterior to the sternocleidomastoid muscle. A diverticulectomy or diverticulopexy can be performed, though a myotomy of the proximal and distal thyropharyngeus and cricopharyngeus muscles should always be performed as there is a 16% recurrence rate [7]. The complication of mediastinitis favors using diverticulopexy and myotomy for small, symptomatic diverticula. In a pexy, the lumen of the diverticulum is suspended in a superior or caudal direction disallowing food particle entry. A large (>5 cm) diverticulum is best treated with ligation and removal of the sac. Endoscopically, the Dohlman procedure is performed by dividing the wall between the diverticulum and esophagus using a laser, bovie cautery, or an endoscopic stapling device. With >3 cm diverticula, symptom relief is the same, and patients have the added benefit of an expedited postoperative course.

Small diverticula in the mid and distal esophagus can forego treatment. Surgery is warranted if larger or with symptoms, and this can be accomplished thorascopically, laparoscopically, or in an open fashion. As these typically lie adjacent to the thoracic spine, a diverticulopexy is sufficient where the sac is sutured to the vertebral fascia [8]. An additional myotomy extending distal to the diverticulum's neck and onto the

LES is often done to relieve the true pathology. With a diverticulectomy, the sac is stapled across its neck, and a myotomy can be performed on the opposite side. An intraoperative Bougie will prevent undue narrowing of the native esophagus. Myotomy is advocated as this will reduce the likelihood of recurrent diverticula [9]. Following diverticulectomy or diverticulopexy, patients can expect to remain in the hospital for 2–3 days.

## Gastroesophageal Reflux Disease and Hiatal Hernia

The most frequent complaint concerning practitioners in this realm is that of heartburn. According to an American Gastroenterological Association Gallup poll, about 50 million Americans experience nighttime heartburn once per week, and just under half report, current remedies do not completely relieve them of their symptoms [10]. All humans experience some normal physiologic reflux, more so when upright and awake. This may occur when swallowing, and the LES relaxes without an oncoming protective food bolus. Pathologic reflux may result with an ineffective LES, inefficient esophageal clearance, and inadequate gastric reservoir. Propulsive forces of the esophagus are relatively weak, being able to overcome only 5–10 grams of weight. Anchoring of the LES is required for efficient propulsion, which is evidenced as reflux when the position is no longer secure.

Based on manometry, a nonfunctioning sphincter has one or more of these characteristics as they fall outside the 2.5 percentile for their given measurements when compared to healthy volunteers [11]:

- Average LES pressure < 6 mmHg
- Average length exposed to the positive pressure environment (abdominal esophagus) <1 cm
- Sphincter length < 2 cm

Unfortunately, pathologic reflux or gastroesophageal reflux disease is a chronic disease and is a major cause of esophagitis. Patients will complain of heartburn, reflux, throat pain, dysphagia, and so forth, though these symptoms may not be specific to GERD. Medical therapy is the mainstay of treatment, and this is often continued throughout a patient's lifetime. With persistent symptoms, workup proceeds with ambulatory pH monitoring and/or esophagogastroduodenoscopy (EGD). When symptoms are refractory to medical therapy or a structural aberrancy is evident, surgical options are pursued as this is the only treatment that can restore the gastroesophageal junction.

Exposure to gastric contents can be detected with a nasogastric probe or capsule (BRAVO ™) that may be clipped to the lower esophageal mucosa. With the capsule, data is transmitted to a monitor worn on the waist, proceeds for 48 h, and is then passed in the stool 1–2 weeks later. These recordings are limited without a pattern or timing of exposure which are necessary to determine the functional deficit resulting in acidic exposure. The cumulative time at pH < 4.0, frequency of episodes, and duration of episodes are combined into a calculated score which is referenced against a normal distribution. Given this, esophageal pH monitoring carries a 96% sensitivity and specificity and is considered the gold standard for diagnosing GERD [11].

There exist several endoluminal and surgical options for GERD, all of which work to functionally reestablish the natural gastroesophageal junction barrier. As there is no incision involved or need to establish pneumoperitoneum, these can be performed under conscious sedation rather than general anesthesia. Endoluminal approaches include suturing or plicating at the GE junction using one of the numerous devices such as EsophyX®, EndoCinch, and the NDO full-thickness plicator. A systematic review of 33 studies involving seven different endoscopic procedures concluded there was insufficient evidence to establish their safety and efficacy, particularly in the long term [12]. The most common of these, the EsophyX, can be performed in 60–90 min and has a cure rate, meaning symptom reduction and discontinued use of PPIs of 56% [13]. Alternatively, radiofrequency energy to the lower esophageal sphincter producing scarring which theoretically stiffens the LES prevents GERD was FDA approved in 2000. Noar and colleagues showed 72% of patients experienced normalization of symptoms immediately and at 10-year follow-up based on a validated questionnaire that assesses current satisfaction and overall heartburn severity [14].

Surgically, the Nissen fundoplication, a 360° wrapping of the gastric fundus around the esophagus to recreate the LES, was first described in the 1950s. This may be approached open or laparoscopically, with the latter being considered the surgical standard for GERD surgical treatment [15]. Several modifications of the original Nissen fundoplication now exist and including re-approximating the diaphragmatic crus or using of a biological mesh reinforcement. Reducing the extent of fundus wrap such as in the Toupet (posterior 180°–270°) and Dor (anterior 180°) fundoplications allows for treatment to be tailored to the patient's needs. Further, without sufficient intra-abdominal esophagus, tubularizing the proximal stomach (Fig. 5.2) prior to fundoplication may be required and referred to as a Collis gastroplasty.

Most recently, there now exists an implantable device, magnetic sphincter augmentation consisting of titanium magnetic band of individually linked beads that restores the lower esophageal sphincter function. This is commercially known as the LINX device (Fig. 5.3). A prospective clinical trial involving 100 patients showed normalization of esophageal acid exposure or a 50% or greater reduction in exposure at 1 year in 64% of patients [16]. Further studies have demonstrated equivocal relief of symptoms to that of LNF with a decrease in being unable to belch [17, 18]. Current short-term results are promising, though robust long-term studies are scarce. In a recent clinical trial including 85 patients followed over 5 years, no device erosions, migrations, malfunctions, or new safety concerns occurred, and participants subjectively responded with a dramatic decrease in GERD symptomatology [19].

Following open surgery, diet will commence with clear liquids and progress after the resumption of bowel function, which can be expected on postoperative day 3 or 4. Patients can expect to go home on day 5. However, with the advent of laparoscopy and principles of minimally invasive surgery, patients undergoing a laparoscopic

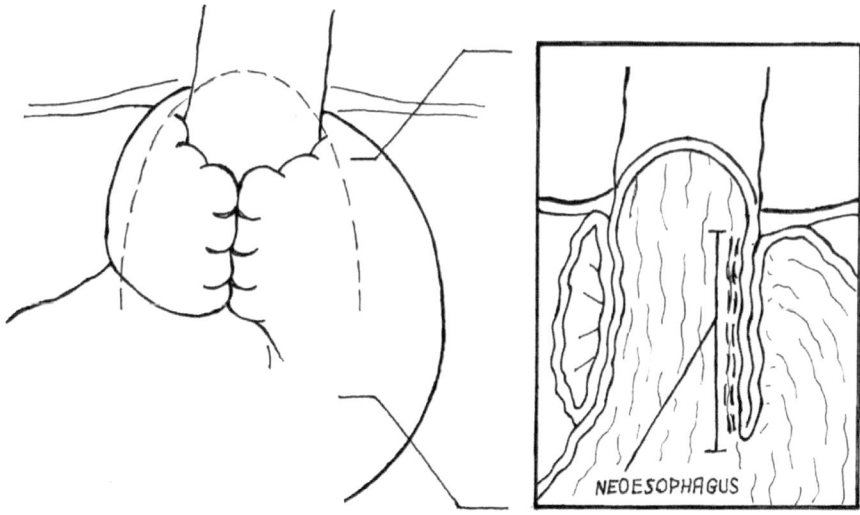

**Fig. 5.2** Nissen fundoplication with Collis gastroplasty

**Fig. 5.3** LINX device

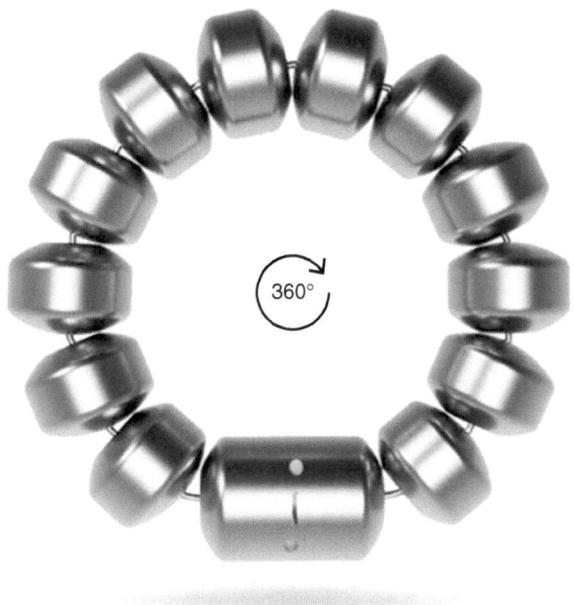

Nissen fundoplication or LINX procedure will typically be started on a liquid diet immediately after surgery and plan for discharge the following day. This surgical approach has dramatically changed the length of stay and patient's return to normal function for those with gastroesophageal reflux disease treated surgically.

# Esophageal Perforation

The esophagus may perforate due to a number of processes ranging from Boerhaave syndrome, trauma, tumor erosion, foreign body ingestion, or iatrogenic causes. A patient presenting to the emergency room will likely have chest neck or throat pain with findings of crepitus on exam. Oral contrast CT or barium swallow study is diagnostic. Mortality from perforation is upward of 30% [11], which can be improved through early recognition and initiation of treatment geared toward source control, i.e., broad-spectrum antibiotics and drainage. Management is based on surgeon judgment and experience as most of the literature is based on retrospective studies. Some base the decision to operate on extent of time of perforation and initiation of treatment, extent of pleural or mediastinal contamination, and the patient's overall clinical picture with contained perforations without overwhelming sepsis treated conservatively or endoscopically with a stent [20, 21]. When due to stricture or tumor, surgical repair with definitive treatment is more appropriate [21, 22]. A study from the University of Pittsburgh Medical Center retrospectively assessed outcomes, and authors were able to devise a scoring system to help stratify patients based on whether or not they undergo surgery. They found patients with lower clinical scores (2 or less) based on factors in Table 5.1 had worse outcomes if they underwent surgery [20].

Options for surgical repair, when indicated, include primary repair and drainage, esophageal resection, or in extreme cases, esophageal exclusion and [22]. A cervical esophagus injury may be contained by surrounding structures and is generally better tolerated. Approach is via a left cervical incision followed by primary repair and drainage. A thoracic injury warrants thoracotomy, right if mid or proximal esophagus, left if distal. Likewise, injury in the abdomen requires celiotomy. Primary repair with a two-layered anastomosis is the goal, though due to the overwhelming

**Table 5.1** Clinical severity score based on Abbas, 2009

| Variable | Score (range 1–3) |
| --- | --- |
| Age >75 years | 1 |
| Tachycardia >100 beats/min | 1 |
| Leukocytosis >10,000 WBC/ml | 1 |
| Pleural effusion (on CXR or CT) | 1 |
| Fever >38.5°C | 2 |
| Noncontained leak (on CT or barium swallow) | 2 |
| Respiratory compromise (respiratory rate >30, mechanical ventilation) | 2 |
| Time to diagnosis >24 h | 2 |
| Cancer | 3 |
| Hypotension | 3 |
| Total potential score | 18 |

Data from [6]
*CT* computed tomography, *CXR* chest x-ray, *WBC* white blood cell

contamination, healing of tissues in that environment may not be possible and an esophagectomy with cervical anastomosis or diversion altogether may be required. In this case, a jejunal feeding tube is also indicated. Primary repair can be reinforced with intercostal muscle, pleural, or omental pedicled flaps as a means to provide reliable vascular inflow and protection to the healing tissue. It is important to be mindful of the etiology of the perforation during repair as this can impair healing. If due to stricture or tumor, these segments should be resected. If due to a motility disorder such as achalasia, a myotomy should be performed. Postoperative recovery should begin with intensive care focused on continued resuscitative efforts such as intravenous hydration, hemodynamic monitoring, broad-spectrum antibiotics, drain and wound care, and nutritional supplementation.

Foreign body ingestion can lead to perforation if not managed carefully. Timing of treatment is based on the object which was ingestion. Urgent resolution is indicated if there is near or complete obstruction (unable to swallow secretions) or if there is respiratory compromise, if the object is sharp or long, or if there are high-powered magnets or a disk battery [23]. Observation for 12–24 h is permissible as spontaneous passage may occur. Endoscopy under general anesthesia is preferred if the object is lodged in the esophagus for more than 24 h [24]. Using long graspers or special lassoes can aid in retrieval. Otherwise, relaxation and lubrication can aid in gently passing the object into the stomach where it can be removed via gastrostomy.

## Neoplasia

When unchecked, reflux can progress to cancer. Esophageal cancer is the sixth leading cause of death worldwide. Figures 5.4 and 5.5 derived from the World Health Organization GLOBOCAN project demonstrate the worldwide esophageal cancer incidence (blue) and mortality (red) numbers per country. The vast majority of esophageal cancer is either squamous cell carcinoma or adenocarcinoma. The former is more so associated with tobacco, alcohol use, and the consumption of hot beverages, while the latter is associated with prolonged symptoms of reflux and the classic progression from metaplasia to dysplasia. From the American Cancer Society, it is estimated that in 2017 about 16,940 new esophageal cancer cases diagnosed (13,360 in men and 3580 in women) and about 15,690 deaths from esophageal cancer (12,720 in men and 2970 in women) with the incidence of adenocarcinoma on the rise [25].

## *Benign Disease*

Many of the benign tumors of the esophagus are rare and described mainly as case reports in the literature. Depending on size, most of these are safely managed with endoscopic techniques. Granular cell tumors (GCT) are neural ectodermal in origin

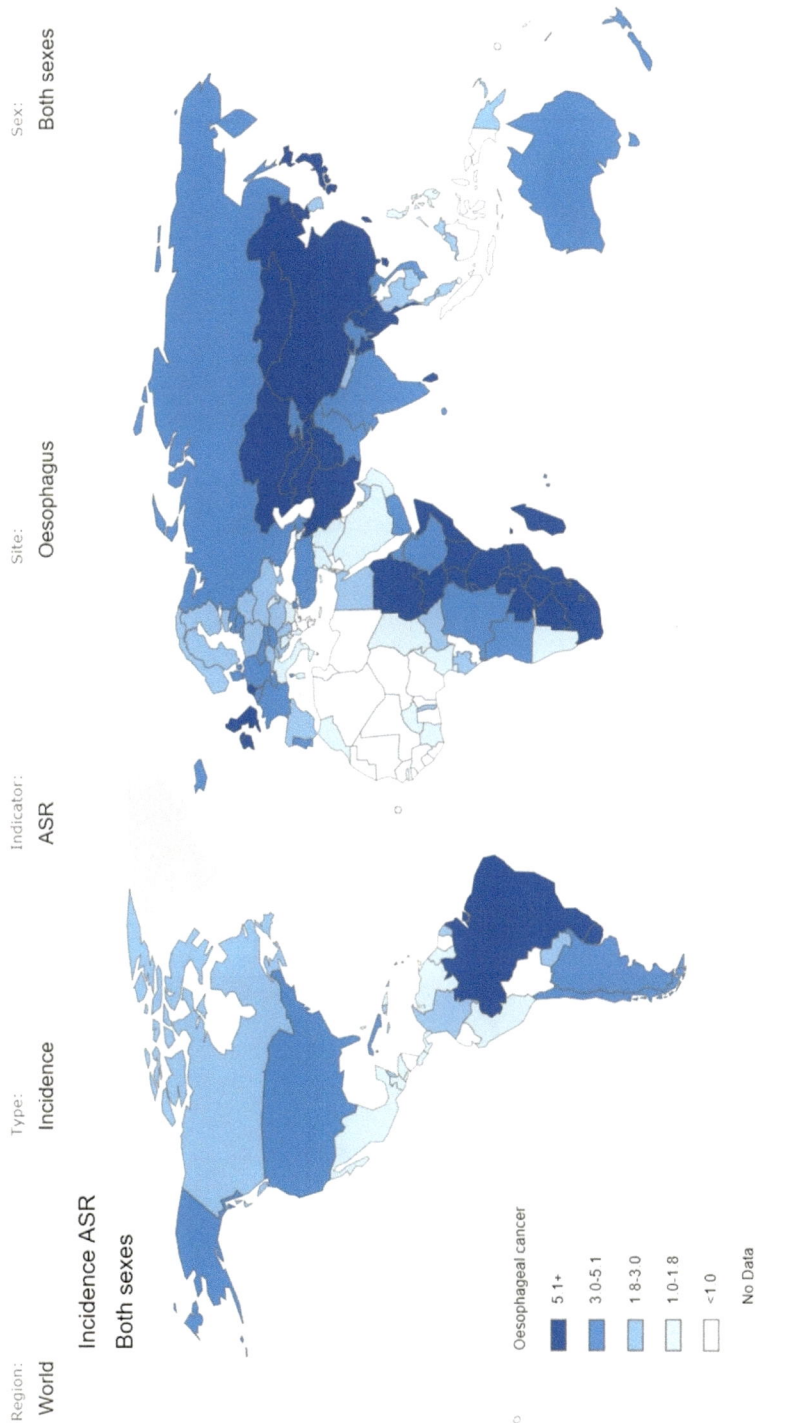

**Fig. 5.4** Esophageal cancer incidence

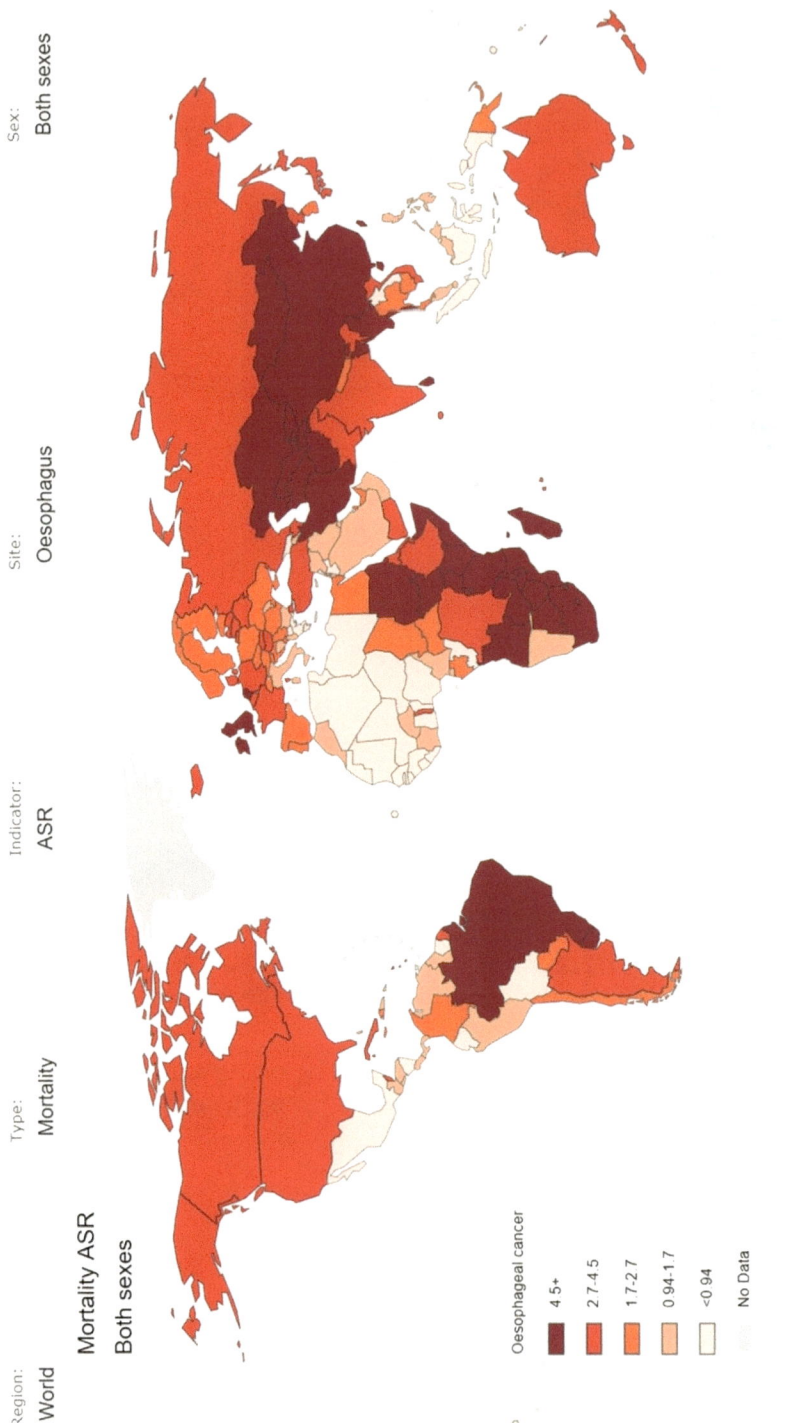

**Fig. 5.5** Esophageal cancer mortality

and are most commonly found in the distal third of the esophagus and are adequately diagnosed with EUS [26]. Fibrovascular polyps are soft tissue tumors and are found mostly in the cervical esophagus. These may present as dysphagia or even airway obstruction. Leiomyomas are the most common benign tumors of the esophagus and are mostly found in the mid to distal esophagus in the muscularis propria. These can be safely enucleated laparoscopically or thoracoscopically without removing parts of the esophagus, with a higher risk of perforation if previously biopsied [27, 28].

## *Biopsy*

The most common presenting symptom for esophageal cancer is dysphagia, and for this, patients will usually undergo barium swallow where a filling defect may be visualized. However, cancer may present only as a plaque, ulceration, or small nodule that would not be evident on barium swallow. Symptoms of weight loss or prolonged reflux should prompt esophagogastroduodenoscopy (EGD) with biopsy. Biopsy is the only definitive means to make a diagnosis. In 1982, Graham et al. established that with greater than seven biopsy samples yields more than 98% of diagnoses [29]. The Seattle biopsy protocol developed by the American College of Gastroenterology is employed if Barrett's esophagus is suspected. Here, four biopsies spaced 2 cm apart should be obtained with particular attention paid to the squamocolumnar junction as most tumors occur within 2 cm to here (Fig. 5.6) [30].

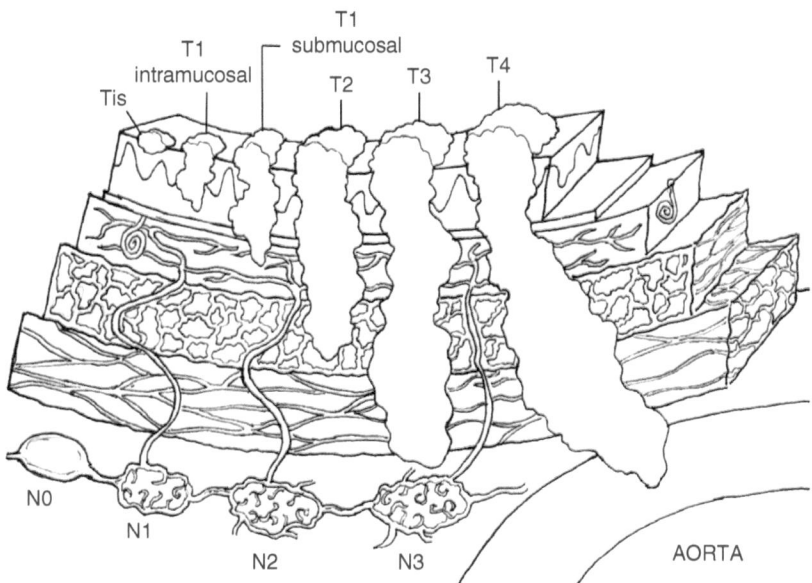

**Fig. 5.6** Depth of tumor invasion by layer and nodal involvement

Once the diagnosis of dysplasia is established, the patient should complete a full workup to stage the disease. This begins with, CT of the chest, abdomen, and pelvis, and 18F-fluorodeoxyglucose positron emission tomography (FDG-PET), or integrated PET-CT, to assess for metastatic disease. If confined to the esophagus and surrounding tissue, endoscopic ultrasound (EUS) is required to determine locoregional staging by gleaning layer of tissue invasion as well as providing the ability to sample surrounding lymph nodes. Staging is currently based on the Union for International Cancer Control (UICC) and the American Joint Committee on Cancer (AJCC) 7th edition, though the 8th edition will begin implementation January 1, 2018. In addition to the already established clinical and pathologic staging systems, newly included in the 8th edition is pathologic staging specifically post-neoadjuvant chemotherapy. This is based on patients experiencing markedly different survivorship when comparing surgery with versus without neoadjuvant chemotherapy [31].

Due to the relatively low incidence in the USA, screening is not cost-effective, and most esophageal cancers are discovered at later stages. Unfortunately, when a patient starts to experience dysphagia, their tumor may already be transmural or T3, with a 77% having nodal metastases [32]. In short, pathology ranging from high-grade dysplasia (HGD) to those confined to the muscularis mucosa (T1a) can be treated with less invasive endoscopic approaches. Locally advanced tumors (T3 tumors or T2 tumors with nodal involvement) require multimodality therapy. Stage IV disease requires systemic or palliative therapy. Distant metastatic disease remains as the main cause of death in patients with esophageal cancer.

Endoscopic mucosal resection (EMR), endoscopic submucosal dissection (ESD), and endoscopic ablation are the treatments of choice for pathology confined to the muscularis mucosa. In a retrospective review of 58 patients with superficial adenocarcinoma of the GEJ, the rates of en bloc resection and curative resection using ESD were 100% and 79%, respectively [33]. However, the rate of perforation after EMR or ESD has been reported up to 5% [34]. Another drawback is the inability for nodal resection. With tumors involving the deepest third of the submucosa, i.e., those that may be considered for ESD, 54% will involve metastases to lymph nodes [35]. Ablative techniques come into play for dysplastic Barrett's esophagus or following endoscopic resection. In an RCT of 127 patients, complete eradication of low-grade and high-grade dysplasia was seen in 90.5% and 81.0%, respectively [36]. Alternatively, ablation may be combined with and follow EMR or ESD 4–12 weeks after the resection site has healed [34].

## Multimodal Therapy

Surgery has been the mainstay of treatment for esophageal cancer T1b and beyond, though outcomes have been poor with 5-year survival estimated at 43% for localized disease [37]. In light of this, pursuit of multimodal therapy has been relentless, and as a result, the role of surgery as a single-modality treatment has decreased. In 2012, the CROSS group showed preoperative chemoradiotherapy improved survival in patients with resectable esophageal cancer. Specifically, complete resection (R0) was achieved in 92% of patients in the chemoradiotherapy-surgery group versus 69% in the surgery-only group (P < 0.001). Importantly, there were no significant differences in postoperative complications, and median overall survival was nearly double, 49.4 months in the chemoradiotherapy-surgery group versus 24.0 months in the surgery-only group [38].

When considering both squamous cell carcinoma and adenocarcinoma, there is strong evidence demonstrating a survival benefit with neoadjuvant chemoradiotherapy or chemotherapy over surgery alone [39]. A current Cochrane review, however, showed the addition of esophagectomy following chemoradiation for locally advanced disease did not change survival much at all, noting this was exclusive for squamous cell carcinoma [40]. A selective resection strategy has also been, meaning proceed with surgical resection only in patients with an incomplete response to neoadjuvant chemoradiation. This approach increased survival among patients with residual disease following neoadjuvant therapy who then went on to resection, compared to those who did not [41].

## Preoperative

Patient selection for surgical esophagectomy is critical in reducing perioperative morbidity and mortality. Cardiorespiratory status and ASA classification should be evaluated to determine if a patient is a good operative candidate and tolerate the stress of this major and relatively lengthy operation.

Patients with esophageal cancer are prone to malnutrition due to dysphagia, decreased appetite, and side effects of neoadjuvant chemoradiation [42]. Using a Japanese nationwide web-based database that included over 5000 patients who underwent esophagectomy, Takeuchi et al. elucidated factors such as smoking within 1 year before surgery, and weight loss more than 10% within 6 months before surgery was associated with 30-day operative mortality [43]. Further studies have shown active smoking and excessive alcohol consumption were linked with the occurrence of severe complications, and some have adopted a requirement that asks patients to discontinue smoking for at least 6 weeks as this has been shown to increase rates of pneumonia [44, 45]. Moderate or severe malnutrition is an independent risk factor for severe morbidity prior to esophagectomy, and assessments using serum albumin, cholesterol, and total lymphocyte count can clue practitioners into a patient's baseline nutritional status as a means to predict postoperative complications [46, 47].

Strategies to mitigate this include optimization of nutritional status using oral dietary supplement have resulted in fewer postoperative infections, shorter hospitalization, and improved 6-month survival [48]. Other groups have sought placement of a feeding jejunostomy tube laparoscopically, prior to esophagectomy. This is both safe and does not interfere with definitive surgical esophageal resection [49]. The dictum of nothing per orem after midnight is mostly a result of a theoretically increased risk of aspiration during intubation. Interestingly, when not fluid restricted preoperatively, patients are found to have lower gastric content volumes, and there is a lack of evidence suggesting a shortened fluid fast results in increased aspiration [50]. The findings of this Cochrane review led to advocating for preoperative carbohydrate drinks to attenuate the surgical stress response and hasten discharge and the recommendation of a 6 h solid food fast and 2 h liquid fast [51].

## Esophagectomy Technique

Goals of surgery include complete tumor removal (R0 resection) including associated lymph nodes while remaining mindful to maximize the patient's postoperative quality of life and minimize morbidity and mortality. Options for esophagectomy vary based on approach to tumor resection, location of anastomosis, and conduit. The variety of approaches include transthoracic esophagectomy (TTE) and transhiatal esophagectomy (THE), and several options exist for the pursuit of these in a minimally invasive fashion (MIE). Of note, each involves access to at least two body cavities. Anastomoses can be made either in the chest or in the neck. Reconstruction is based on raising a gastric conduit or using a colon or jejunal interposition if the stomach is unavailable.

TTE, better known as the Ivor Lewis operation, was first described and popularized in the 1940s. Traditionally, this approach employs two incisions, a right thoracotomy and laparotomy. Laparotomy allows for GE dissection and amply nodal harvest, meanwhile thoracotomy permits direct thoracic esophagus dissection and subsequent anastomosis. The McKeown modification of this approach employs a third, left cervical incision to create a side-to-side anastomosis in the neck. THE relies on a transabdominal incision for dissection and a separate cervical incision for the final anastomosis. Increased use of this approach is due to a rise in GEJ adenocarcinoma. The advantage here is avoidance of the morbidity associated with a thoracotomy incision as well as the devastating complication of a thoracic anastomotic leak and subsequent mediastinitis. An anastomotic leak in the neck is managed with simply opening the wound. Disadvantage with this approach includes blunt dissection of the esophagus from the distal trachea to subcarinal (5–10 cm) which reduces the surgeon's ability to control bleeding structures, decreased quality of lymphadenectomy [8], and increased swallowing morbidity and recurrent laryngeal nerve injury with the cervical incision [52, 53]. Having said this, contraindications for a THE include mid to upper esophageal cancers and previous thoracotomy as there may be disruption of the safe paraesophageal space used in the blunt dissection.

MIE uses thoracoscopy and laparoscopy to reduce the physical burden of large incisions without compromising the goals of the operation. A "hybrid" operation may involve a minimally invasive approach combined with an open incision elsewhere. For example, a right thoracoscopic approach can allow for mobilization of the esophagus without morbidity of a thoracotomy incision, and this can be combined with a laparotomy. Totally minimally invasive esophagectomy avoids any thoracotomy or laparotomy incision, and the anastomosis can be intrathoracic or cervical. Figures 5.7 and 5.8 show an example of typical trocar placement for the thoracic and abdominal portions of the operation, respectively.

The minimally invasive approach has demonstrable improvements compared to using open incisions. The TIME trial was directly compared both in a randomized controlled fashion. Investigators showed a significantly decreased rate of pulmonary infection with the minimally invasive approach and no difference in disease-free and overall survival at 3-year follow-up [54, 55]. In a study of 20 meta-analyses, which included 4 RCTs, authors determined there was a significant decrease in operative blood loss, reduction in respiratory complications, and better overall survival with MIE versus open esophagectomy [56]. Furthermore, a long-term health-related quality of life study demonstrated greater scores for pain and constipation with open surgery compared to a thoracoscopically assisted approach [57]. MIE is also associated with decreased median length of stay, leak rate, and wound infection and is safe following neoadjuvant chemoradiation [58]. When examining minimally invasive TTE and THE, the TTE approach results in significantly decreased serious (Clavien-Dindo 3, 4, or 5) complications postoperatively [59].

**Fig. 5.7** Thoracic trocar placement

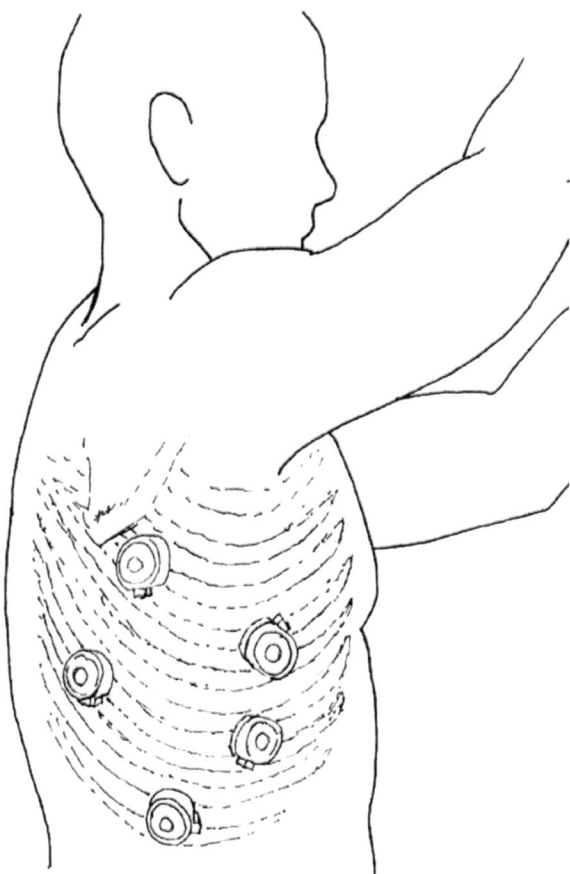

**Fig. 5.8** Abdominal trocar placement

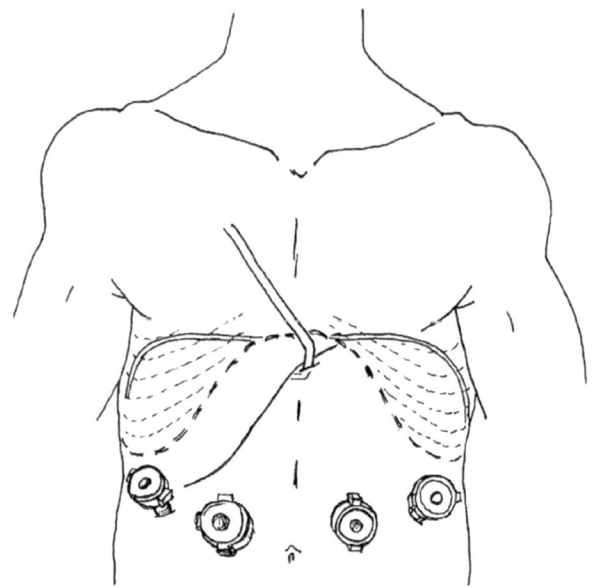

Nodal dissection is an important consideration when distinguishing approaches as this serves two purposes, staging and local control. Ideally, 15–30 nodes should be sent with the esophageal specimen during definitive resection because the pattern of lymphatic spread is quite variable. A large series showed no significant difference in number of nodes harvested with MIE Ivor Lewis, and MIE McKeown [52]. However, Altorki et al. discovered recurrent laryngeal and/or deep cervical nodes occurred in 36% of patients irrespective of cell type (adenocarcinoma 37%, squamous 34%) or location within the esophagus (lower third 32%, middle third 60%) [60].

Lastly, it is not uncommon for patients to be NPO status for several days to weeks postoperatively, depending on the surgeon's practice. If not placed preoperatively, many surgeons advocate placement of a feeding jejunostomy at the time of definitive resection to enhance nutritional status in patient that is more likely than not to be malnourished. To contrast, Fenton et al. described a retrospective cohort of feeding jejunostomy tubes placed at the time of esophageal surgery where 76.9% of patients had returned to oral intake before discharge (median, 7 days) [61]. Here, logistical regression analysis determined only patients with body mass index less than or equal to 18.5 kg/m² who were more likely to require a feeding JT at discharge.

## Postoperatively

Patients can expect to remain hospitalized for 1–2 weeks following surgery. Given the complexity of surgery, intensive care monitoring is routine for the first day or two after surgery. A nasogastric decompression with the tip beyond the anastomosis is usually kept to low suction and remains until resumption of bowel function, usually day 3–5. Decompression may decrease leak rate as well as reduce respiratory complications [62]. Diet may be advanced after this as early enteral feeding following all gastrointestinal surgery is not associated with increased anastomotic dehiscence and can reduce infection and length of hospitalization [63]. Some advocate employing a comprehensive swallowing evaluation prior to starting oral feeds to reduce occult aspiration and ensuing pneumonia; this is routine in our practice [64]. This may also shed light on swallowing mechanics in the assessment of delayed gastric emptying, reflux, or dumping syndrome.

When the stomach conduit is elevated to the thorax, it is now in a negative pressure environment. In a cancer operation, the vagus nerve is rarely spared, also contributing to aberrancy in normal motility. Patients will no longer have the diaphragmatic contribution to prevent reflux. Resection of the fundus diminishes signaling factors for receptive expansion. The interplay of these changes can lead to delayed gastric emptying, an occurrence reported in 10–20% of patients' post-esophagectomy [65–67]. Patients may have symptoms of nausea, vomiting, bloating, early satiety, and distension, though these are hardly specific and may also signal anastomotic stricture. Some advocate the use of promotility agents such as metoclopramide or erythromycin to start. Trials of botulism injection in the pylorus have also demonstrated short-term promise [68, 69]. Myotomy, pyloroplasty, or pyloric balloon dilatation can prevent (when done during primary resection) or treat symptoms [65]. Stricture may occur postoperatively presenting as dysphagia. Early this may result from scar contracture and usually resolves without intervention. If persistent, endoscopic balloon dilation can ameliorate symptoms yet with up to 50% recurrence and need for repeat dilation [70, 71]. Late stricture may signal tumor recurrence and should be pursued with endoscopy or PET/CT.

It is also recommended that at the conclusion of surgery, a drain or chest tube be placed in the ipsilateral pleural space to prevent pulmonary compression and monitor for hemorrhage, leak, or chylothorax. One drain is just as effective as multiple in accomplishing this goal, and the drain may be removed when draining 200 mL per day to reduce pain and length of stay [51]. Practitioners should exercise vigilant monitoring for anastomotic leak, especially if anastomosis is within the thoracic cavity. Clinically, patients may exhibit fever, new onset arrhythmias, or other signs of sepsis such as confusion or hypotension. Laboratory markers such as leukocytosis or lactic acidosis can clue practitioners for an impending or already occurring leak [72]. Routine barium swallow for the detection of a leak is not necessary in all patients as there is low sensitivity (36%) but can be employed if a leak is suspected [73]. Some have advocated the use of postoperative endoscopy to evaluate the resultant conduit [74].

A chylothorax may result if the thoracic duct was inadvertently injured. This is a rare complication seen in <4% of patients but should be expected if chest drains begin to exhibit a brownish or milky fluid [75]. Sampling of the fluid will demonstrate triglyceride concentrations >110 mg/dL. Conservative measures should be initiated promptly. These include initiation of a low-fat, high-protein diet with supplementation of medium-chain fatty acids, or even discontinuing oral intake and providing parenteral nutrition. Effective control is when chest tube drainage reduces to <200–300 mL per day. A marker of 10 mL/kg at day 5 can indicate whether a patient will require surgery [76]. If the leak persists, surgical closure of the thoracic duct may be warranted.

## *Other Malignant Tumors*

The esophagus may harbor several other primary malignancies including gastrointestinal stromal tumor (GIST), sarcoma, small cell carcinoma, and primary melanoma. The incidence of these is certainly dwarfed by that of squamous cell carcinoma and adenocarcinoma. GIST mostly occurs in the stomach and is very rarely found primarily in the esophagus (<1%) [77]. Given the rarity, controversy exists regarding optimal treatment. Enucleation may prohibit achievement of an R0 resection compared to resection. If small, these may be resected with the goal being negative margins. Esophagectomy is recommended if greater than 9 cm [78]. Tyrosine kinase inhibitors (e.g., imatinib) should be added for tumors >3 cm or with high-risk features [79].

## References

1. Leeuwenburgh I, et al. Long-term esophageal cancer risk in patients with primary achalasia: a prospective study. Am J Gastroenterol. 2010;105(10):2144–9. https://doi.org/10.1038/ajg.2010.263.
2. Leite LP, Johnston BT, Barrett J, Castell JA, Castell DO. Ineffective esophageal motility (IEM): the primary finding in patients with nonspecific esophageal motility disorder. Dig Dis Sci. 1997;42(9):1859–65. PubMed PMID: 9331148.
3. Code CF, Schlegel JF, Kelley ML Jr, et al. Hypertensive gastroesophageal sphincter. Proc Staff Meet Mayo Clin. 1960;35:391–9.
4. Teitelbaum EN, Dunst CM, Reavis KM, Sharata AM, Ward MA, DeMeester SR, Swanström LL. Clinical outcomes five years after POEM for treatment of primary esophageal motility disorders. Surg Endosc. 2018;32(1):421–7. https://doi.org/10.1007/s00464-017-5699-2.
5. Schlottmann F, Luckett DJ, Fine J, Shaheen NJ, Patti MG. Laparoscopic Heller myotomy versus peroral endoscopic myotomy (POEM) for achalasia: a systematic review and meta-analysis. Ann Surg. 2018;267(3):451–60. https://doi.org/10.1097/SLA.0000000000002311.
6. Gutschow CA, Hamoir M, Rombaux P, Otte JB, Goncette L, Collard JM. Management of pharyngoesophageal (Zenker's) diverticulum: which technique? Ann Thorac Surg. 2002;74(5):1677–82; discussion 1682–3.
7. Skinner KA, Zuckerbraun L. Recurrent Zenker's diverticulum: treatment with cricopharyngeal myotomy. Am Surg. 1998;64:192–5.
8. Nehra D, Lord RV, DeMeester TR, Theisen J, Peters JH, Crookes PF, Bremner CG. Physiologic basis for the treatment of epiphrenic diverticulum. Ann Surg. 2002;235(3):346–54. PubMed PMID: 11882756; PubMed Central PMCID: PMC1422440.
9. Shaker R, et al. Nighttime heartburn is an under-appreciated clinical problem that impacts sleep and daytime function: the results of a gallup survey conducted on behalf of the American

Gastroenterological Association. Am J Gastroenterol. 2003;98(7):1487–93. https://doi.org/10.1111/j.1572-0241.2003.07531.x.

10. Chen D, Barber C, McLoughlin P, Thavaneswaran P, Jamieson GG, Maddern GJ. Systematic review of endoscopic treatments for gastro-oesophageal reflux disease. Br J Surg. 2009;96(2):128–36. https://doi.org/10.1002/bjs.6440. Review. PubMed PMID: 19160349.

11. Cadière GB, Buset M, Muls V, Rajan A, Rösch T, Eckardt AJ, Weerts J, Bastens B, Costamagna G, Marchese M, Louis H, Mana F, Sermon F, Gawlicka AK, Daniel MA, Devière J. Antireflux transoral incisionless fundoplication using EsophyX: 12-month results of a prospective multi-center study. World J Surg. 2008;32(8):1676–88. https://doi.org/10.1007/s00268-008-9594-9. PubMed PMID: 18443855; PubMed Central PMCID: PMC2490723.

12. Noar M, Squires P, Noar E, Lee M. Long-term maintenance effect of radiofrequency energy delivery for refractory GERD: a decade later. Surg Endosc. 2014;28(8):2323–33. https://doi.org/10.1007/s00464-014-3461-6. Epub 2014 Feb 22. PubMed PMID: 24562599.

13. Salminen P. The laparoscopic Nissen fundoplication – a better operation? Surgeon. 2009;4:224–7.

14. Ganz RA, Peters JH, Horgan S, et al. Esophageal sphincter device for gastroesophageal reflux disease. N Engl J Med. 2013;368:719–27.

15. Reynolds JL, Zehetner J, Wu P, Shah S, Bildzukewicz N, Lipham JC. Laparoscopic magnetic sphincter augmentation vs laparoscopic Nissen fundoplication: a matched-pair analysis of 100 patients. J Am Coll Surg. 2015;221(1):123–8. https://doi.org/10.1016/j.jamcollsurg.2015.02.025. Epub 2015 Mar 5. PubMed PMID: 26095560.

16. Skubleny D, Switzer NJ, Dang J, Gill RS, Shi X, de Gara C, Birch DW, Wong C, Hutter MM, Karmali S. LINX® magnetic esophageal sphincter augmentation versus Nissen fundoplication for gastroesophageal reflux disease: a systematic review and meta-analysis. Surg Endosc. 2017;31(8):3078–84. https://doi.org/10.1007/s00464-016-5370-3. Epub 2016 Dec 15. PubMed PMID: 27981382.

17. Ganz RA, Edmundowicz SA, Taiganides PA, Lipham JC, Smith CD, DeVault KR, Horgan S, Jacobsen G, Luketich JD, Smith CC, Schlack-Haerer SC, Kothari SN, Dunst CM, Watson TJ, Peters J, Oelschlager BK, Perry KA, Melvin S, Bemelman WA, Smout AJ, Dunn D. Long-term Outcomes of Patients Receiving a Magnetic Sphincter Augmentation Device for Gastroesophageal Reflux. Clin Gastroenterol Hepatol. 2016;14(5):671–7. https://doi.org/10.1016/j.cgh.2015.05.028. Epub 2015 Jun 2. PubMed PMID: 26044316.

18. Abbas G, Schuchert MJ, Pettiford BL, Pennathur A, Landreneau J, Landreneau J, Luketich JD, Landreneau RJ. Contemporaneous management of esophageal perforation. Surgery. 2009;146(4):749–55. https://doi.org/10.1016/j.surg.2009.06.058; discussion 755–6. PubMed PMID: 19789035.

19. Felmly LM, Kwon H, Denlinger CE, Klapper JA. Esophageal perforation: a common clinical problem with many different management options. Am Surg. 2017;83(8):911–7. PubMed PMID: 28822401.

20. Sepesi B, Raymond DP, Peters JH. Esophageal perforation: surgical, endoscopic and medical management strategies. Curr Opin Gastroenterol. 2010;26(4):379–83.

21. Gilger, MA, et al. Foreign bodies of the esophagus and gastrointestinal tract in children. UpToDate, 3 Mar. 2017, www.uptodate.com/contents/foreign-bodies-of-the-esophagus-and-gastrointestinal-tract-in-children#H6

22. Soprano JV, Fleisher GR, Mandl KD. The spontaneous passage of esophageal coins in children. Arch Pediatr Adolesc Med. 1999;153(10):1073–6. PubMed PMID: 10520616.

23. Key Statistics for Esophageal Cancer. American Cancer Society, www.cancer.org/cancer/esophagus-cancer/about/key-statistics.html

24. Chen WS, Zheng XL, Jin L, Pan XJ, Ye MF. Novel diagnosis and treatment of esophageal granular cell tumor: report of 14 cases and review of the literature. Ann Thorac Surg. 2014;97(1):296–302. https://doi.org/10.1016/j.athoracsur.2013.08.042. Epub 2013 Oct 17. Review. PubMed PMID: 24140217.

25. Ben-David K, Alvarez J, Rossidis G, Desart K, Caranasos T, Hochwald S. Thoracoscopic and laparoscopic enucleation of esophageal leiomyomas. J Gastrointest Surg. 2015;19(7):1350–4. https://doi.org/10.1007/s11605-015-2817-0. Epub 2015 Apr 14. PubMed PMID: 25868871.

26. Bonavina L, Segalin A, Rosati R, Pavanello M, Peracchia A. Surgical therapy of esophageal leiomyoma. J Am Coll Surg. 1995;181(3):257–62. PubMed PMID: 7670685.
27. Graham DY, Schwartz JT, Cain GD, Gyorkey F. Prospective evaluation of biopsy number in the diagnosis of esophageal and gastric carcinoma. Gastroenterology. 1982;82(2):228–31. PubMed PMID: 7054024.
28. Sampliner RE. Practice guidelines on the diagnosis, surveillance, and therapy of Barrett's esophagus. The Practice Parameters Committee of the American College of Gastroenterology. Am J Gastroenterol. 1998;93(7):1028–32. PubMed PMID: 9672324.
29. Edge SB, Byrd DR, Compton CC, et al., editors. American joint committee on cancer staging manual. 7th ed. New York: Springer; 2010. p. 103.
30. Rice TW, Zuccaro G Jr, Adelstein DJ, Rybicki LA, Blackstone EH, Goldblum JR. Esophageal carcinoma: depth of tumor invasion is predictive of regional lymph node status. Ann Thorac Surg. 1998;65(3):787–92. PubMed PMID: 9527214.
31. Rice TW, et al. 8th edition AJCC/UICC staging of cancers of the esophagus and esophagogastric junction: application to clinical practice. Ann Cardiothorac Surg. 2017;6(2):119–30. https://doi.org/10.21037/acs.2017.03.14. PubMed PMID: 28447000.
32. di Pietro M, Canto MI, Fitzgerald RC. Endoscopic management of early adenocarcinoma and squamous cell carcinoma of the esophagus-screening, diagnosis, and therapy. Gastroenterology. 2017;pii: S0016-5085(17)35973-5. doi: https://doi.org/10.1053/j.gastro.2017.07.041. PubMed PMID: 28778650.
33. Gockel I, Sgourakis G, Lyros O, Polotzek U, Schimanski CC, Lang H, Hoppo T, Jobe BA. Risk of lymph node metastasis in submucosal esophageal cancer: a review of surgically resected patients. Expert Rev Gastroenterol Hepatol. 2011;5(3):371–84. https://doi.org/10.1586/egh.11.33. Review. PubMed PMID: 21651355.
34. Shaheen NJ, Sharma P, Overholt BF, Wolfsen HC, Sampliner RE, Wang KK, Galanko JA, Bronner MP, Goldblum JR, Bennett AE, Jobe BA, Eisen GM, Fennerty MB, Hunter JG, Fleischer DE, Sharma VK, Hawes RH, Hoffman BJ, Rothstein RI, Gordon SR, Mashimo H, Chang KJ, Muthusamy VR, Edmundowicz SA, Spechler SJ, Siddiqui AA, Souza RF, Infantolino A, Falk GW, Kimmey MB, Madanick RD, Chak A, Lightdale CJ. Radiofrequency ablation in Barrett's esophagus with dysplasia. N Engl J Med. 2009;360(22):2277–88. https://doi.org/10.1056/NEJMoa0808145. PubMed PMID: 19474425.
35. Treating Esophageal Cancer by Stage. American Cancer Society, https://www.cancer.org/cancer/esophagus-cancer/treating/by-stage.html
36. van Hagen P, Hulshof MC, van Lanschot JJ, Steyerberg EW, van Berge Henegouwen MI, Wijnhoven BP, Richel DJ, Nieuwenhuijzen GA, Hospers GA, Bonenkamp JJ, Cuesta MA, Blaisse RJ, Busch OR, ten Kate FJ, Creemers GJ, Punt CJ, Plukker JT, Verheul HM, Spillenaar Bilgen EJ, van Dekken H, van der Sangen MJ, Rozema T, Biermann K, Beukema JC, Piet AH, van Rij CM, Reinders JG, Tilanus HW, van der Gaast A, CROSS Group. Preoperative chemoradiotherapy for esophageal or junctional cancer. N Engl J Med. 2012;366(22):2074–84. https://doi.org/10.1056/NEJMoa1112088. PubMed PMID: 22646630.
37. Sjoquist KM, Burmeister BH, Smithers BM, Zalcberg JR, Simes RJ, Barbour A, Gebski V, Australasian Gastro-Intestinal Trials Group. Survival after neoadjuvant chemotherapy or chemoradiotherapy for resectable oesophageal carcinoma: an updated meta-analysis. Lancet Oncol. 2011;12(7):681–92. https://doi.org/10.1016/S1470-2045(11)70142-5. Epub 2011 Jun 16. PubMed PMID: 21684205.
38. Vellayappan BA, Soon YY, Ku GY, Leong CN, Lu JJ, Tey JCS. Chemoradiotherapy versus chemoradiotherapy plus surgery for esophageal cancer. Cochrane Database Syst Rev 2017;8:CD010511. doi: https://doi.org/10.1002/14651858.CD010511.pub2.
39. Swisher SG, Moughan J, Komaki RU, Ajani JA, Wu TT, Hofstetter WL, Konski AA, Willett CG. Final results of NRG oncology RTOG 0246: an organ-preserving selective resection strategy in esophageal cancer patients treated with definitive chemoradiation. J Thorac Oncol. 2017;12(2):368–74. https://doi.org/10.1016/j.jtho.2016.10.002. Epub 2016 Oct 8. PubMed PMID: 27729298; PubMed Central PMCID: PMC5263046.

40. Knight CE. Nutrition considerations in esophagectomy patients. Nutr Clin Pract. 2008;23(5):521–8. https://doi.org/10.1177/0884533608323427. Review. PubMed PMID: 18849557.

41. Takeuchi H, Miyata H, Gotoh M, Kitagawa Y, Baba H, Kimura W, Tomita N, Nakagoe T, Shimada M, Sugihara K, Mori M. A risk model for esophagectomy using data of 5354 patients included in a Japanese nationwide web-based database. Ann Surg. 2014;260(2):259–66. https://doi.org/10.1097/SLA.0000000000000644. PubMed PMID: 24743609.

42. Ben-David K, Rossidis G, Zlotecki RA, Grobmyer SR, Cendan JC, Sarosi GA, Hochwald SN. Minimally invasive esophagectomy is safe and effective following neoadjuvant chemoradiation therapy. Ann Surg Oncol. 2011;18(12):3324–9. https://doi.org/10.1245/s10434-011-1702-7. Epub 2011 Apr 9. PubMed PMID: 21479689.

43. Mantziari S, Hübner M, Demartines N, Schäfer M. Impact of preoperative risk factors on morbidity after esophagectomy: is there room for improvement? World J Surg. 2014;38(11):2882–90. https://doi.org/10.1007/s00268-014-2686-9. PubMed PMID: 25002245.

44. Nozoe T, Kimura Y, Ishida M, Saeki H, Korenaga D, Sugimachi K. Correlation of pre-operative nutritional condition with post-operative complications in surgical treatment for oesophageal carcinoma. Eur J Surg Oncol. 2002;28(4):396–400. PubMed PMID: 12099649.

45. Yoshida N, Baba Y, Shigaki H, Harada K, Iwatsuki M, Kurashige J, Sakamoto Y, Miyamoto Y, Ishimoto T, Kosumi K, Tokunaga R, Imamura Y, Ida S, Hiyoshi Y, Watanabe M, Baba H. Preoperative nutritional assessment by controlling nutritional status (CONUT) is useful to estimate postoperative morbidity after esophagectomy for esophageal cancer. World J Surg. 2016;40(8):1910–7. https://doi.org/10.1007/s00268-016-3549-3. PubMed PMID: 27220507.

46. Kubota K, Kuroda J, Yoshida M, Okada A, Deguchi T, Kitajima M. Preoperative oral supplementation support in patients with esophageal cancer. J Nutr Health Aging. 2014;18(4):437–40. https://doi.org/10.1007/s12603-014-0018-2. PubMed PMID: 24676327.

47. Ben-David K, Kim T, Caban AM, Rossidis G, Rodriguez SS, Hochwald SN. Pre-therapy laparoscopic feeding jejunostomy is safe and effective in patients undergoing minimally invasive esophagectomy for cancer. J Gastrointest Surg. 2013;17(8):1352–8. https://doi.org/10.1007/s11605-013-2231-4. Epub 2013 May 25. PubMed PMID: 23709367.

48. Brady M, Kinn S, Stuart P. Preoperative fasting for adults to prevent perioperative complications. Cochrane Database Syst Rev. 2003;4:CD004423. Review. PubMed PMID: 14584013.

49. Findlay JM, Gillies RS, Millo J, Sgromo B, Marshall RE, Maynard ND. Enhanced recovery for esophagectomy: a systematic review and evidence-based guidelines. Ann Surg. 2014;259(3):413–31. https://doi.org/10.1097/SLA.0000000000000349. Review. PubMed PMID: 24253135.

50. Luketich JD, Pennathur A, Awais O, Levy RM, Keeley S, Shende M, Christie NA, Weksler B, Landreneau RJ, Abbas G, Schuchert MJ, Nason KS. Outcomes after minimally invasive esophagectomy: review of over 1000 patients. Ann Surg. 2012;256(1):95–103. https://doi.org/10.1097/SLA.0b013e3182590603. PubMed PMID: 22668811; PubMed Central PMCID: PMC4103614.

51. van Workum F, Berkelmans GH, Klarenbeek BR, Nieuwenhuijzen GAP, Luyer MDP, Rosman C. McKeown or Ivor Lewis totally minimally invasive esophagectomy for cancer of the esophagus and gastroesophageal junction: systematic review and meta-analysis. J Thorac Dis. 2017;9(Suppl 8):S826–33. https://doi.org/10.21037/jtd.2017.03.173. PubMed PMID: 28815080; PubMed Central PMCID: PMC5538973.

52. Biere SS, van Berge Henegouwen MI, Maas KW, Bonavina L, Rosman C, Garcia JR, Gisbertz SS, Klinkenbijl JH, Hollmann MW, de Lange ES, Bonjer HJ, van der Peet DL, Cuesta MA. Minimally invasive versus open oesophagectomy for patients with oesophageal cancer: a multicentre, open-label, randomised controlled trial. Lancet. 2012;379(9829):1887–92. https://doi.org/10.1016/S0140-6736(12)60516-9. Epub 2012 May 1. PubMed PMID: 22552194.

53. Straatman J, van der Wielen N, Nieuwenhuijzen GA, Rosman C, Roig J, Scheepers JJ, Cuesta MA, Luyer MD, van Berge Henegouwen MI, van Workum F, Gisbertz SS, van der Peet DL. Techniques and short-term outcomes for total minimally invasive Ivor Lewis esopha-

geal resection in distal esophageal and gastroesophageal junction cancers: pooled data from six European centers. Surg Endosc. 2017;31(1):119–26. https://doi.org/10.1007/s00464-016-4938-2. Epub 2016 Apr 29. PubMed PMID: 27129563; PubMed Central PMCID: PMC5216077.

54. Lv L, Hu W, Ren Y, Wei X. Minimally invasive esophagectomy versus open esophagectomy for esophageal cancer: a meta-analysis. Onco Targets Ther. 2016;9:6751–62. eCollection 2016. PubMed PMID: 27826201; PubMed Central PMCID: PMC5096744.

55. Barbour AP, Cormack OMM, Baker PJ, Hirst J, Krause L, Brosda S, Thomas JM, Blazeby JM, Thomson IG, Gotley DC, Smithers BM. Long-term health-related quality of life following esophagectomy: a nonrandomized comparison of thoracoscopically assisted and open surgery. Ann Surg. 2017;265(6):1158–65. https://doi.org/10.1097/SLA.0000000000001899. PubMed PMID: 27429022.

56. Ben-David K, Sarosi GA, Cendan JC, Howard D, Rossidis G, Hochwald SN. Decreasing morbidity and mortality in 100 consecutive minimally invasive esophagectomies. Surg Endosc. 2012;26(1):162–7. https://doi.org/10.1007/s00464-011-1846-3. Epub 2011 Jul 27. PubMed PMID: 21792712.

57. Brown AM, Pucci MJ, Berger AC, Tatarian T, Evans NR 3rd, Rosato EL, Palazzo F. A standardized comparison of peri-operative complications after minimally invasive esophagectomy: Ivor Lewis versus McKeown. Surg Endosc. 2018;32(1):204–11. https://doi.org/10.1007/s00464-017-5660-4.

58. Altorki N, Kent M, Ferrara C, Port J. Three-field lymph node dissection for squamous cell and adenocarcinoma of the esophagus. Ann Surg. 2002;236(2):177–83. PubMed PMID: 12170022; PubMed Central PMCID: PMC1422563.

59. Fenton JR, Bergeron EJ, Coello M, Welsh RJ, Chmielewski GW. Feeding jejunostomy tubes placed during esophagectomy: are they necessary? Ann Thorac Surg. 2011;92(2):504–11. https://doi.org/10.1016/j.athoracsur.2011.03.101; discussion 511–2. Epub 2011 Jun 24. PubMed PMID: 21704294.

60. Shackcloth MJ, McCarron E, Kendall J, Russell GN, Pennefather SH, Tran J, Page RD. Randomized clinical trial to determine the effect of nasogastric drainage on tracheal acid aspiration following oesophagectomy. Br J Surg. 2006;93(5):547–52. PubMed PMID: 16521172.

61. Lewis SJ, Egger M, Sylvester PA, Thomas S. Early enteral feeding versus "nil by mouth" after gastrointestinal surgery: systematic review and meta-analysis of controlled trials. BMJ. 2001;323(7316):773–6. PubMed PMID: 11588077; PubMed Central PMCID: PMC57351.

62. Berry MF, Atkins BZ, Tong BC, Harpole DH, D'Amico TA, Onaitis MW. A comprehensive evaluation for aspiration after esophagectomy reduces the incidence of postoperative pneumonia. J Thorac Cardiovasc Surg. 2010;140(6):1266–71. https://doi.org/10.1016/j.jtcvs.2010.08.038. Epub 2010 Sep 29. PubMed PMID: 20884018; PubMed Central PMCID: PMC3147296.

63. Lanuti M, DeDelva P, Morse CR, Wright CD, Wain JC, Gaissert HA, Donahue DM, Mathisen DJ. Management of delayed gastric emptying after esophagectomy with endoscopic balloon dilatation of the pylorus. Ann Thorac Surg. 2011;91(4):1019–24. https://doi.org/10.1016/j.athoracsur.2010.12.055. Epub 2011 Feb 2. PubMed PMID: 21292237.

64. Lee HS, Kim MS, Lee JM, Kim SK, Kang KW, Zo JI. Intrathoracic gastric emptying of solid food after esophagectomy for esophageal cancer. Ann Thorac Surg. 2005;80(2):443–7. PubMed PMID: 16039182.

65. Sutcliffe RP, Forshaw MJ, Tandon R, Rohatgi A, Strauss DC, Botha AJ, Mason RC. Anastomotic strictures and delayed gastric emptying after esophagectomy: incidence, risk factors and management. Dis Esophagus. 2008;21:712–7. https://doi.org/10.1111/j.1442-2050.2008.00865.x.

66. Kent MS, Pennathur A, Fabian T, McKelvey A, Schuchert MJ, Luketich JD, Landreneau RJ. A pilot study of botulinum toxin injection for the treatment of delayed gastric emptying following esophagectomy. Surg Endosc. 2007;21(5):754–7. Epub 2007 Feb 16. Erratum in: Surg Endosc. 2007 Nov;21(11):2120. PubMed PMID: 17458616.

67. Martin JT, Federico JA, McKelvey AA, Kent MS, Fabian T. Prevention of delayed gastric emptying after esophagectomy: a single center's experience with botulinum toxin. Ann Thorac

Surg.  2009;87(6):1708–13.  https://doi.org/10.1016/j.athoracsur.2009.01.075;  discussion 1713-4. PubMed PMID: 19463583.

68. Mendelson AH, Small AJ, Agarwalla A, Scott FI, Kochman ML. Esophageal anastomotic strictures: outcomes of endoscopic dilation, risk of recurrence and refractory stenosis, and effect of foreign body removal. Clin Gastroenterol Hepatol. 2015;13(2):263–271.e1. https://doi.org/10.1016/j.cgh.2014.07.010. Epub 2014 Jul 11. PubMed PMID: 25019695; PubMed Central PMCID: PMC4289652.

69. Park JY, Song HY, Kim JH, Park JH, Na HK, Kim YH, Park SI. Benign anastomotic strictures after esophagectomy: long-term effectiveness of balloon dilation and factors affecting recurrence in 155 patients. AJR Am J Roentgenol. 2012;198(5):1208–13. https://doi.org/10.2214/AJR.11.7608. PubMed PMID: 22528915.

70. Ip B, Ng KT, Packer S, Paterson-Brown S, Couper GW. High serum lactate as an adjunct in the early prediction of anastomotic leak following oesophagectomy. Int J Surg. 2017;46:7–10. https://doi.org/10.1016/j.ijsu.2017.08.027. PubMed PMID: 28803998.

71. Roh S, Iannettoni MD, Keech JC, Bashir M, Gruber PJ, Parekh KR. Role of barium swallow in diagnosing clinically significant anastomotic leak following esophagectomy. Korean J Thorac Cardiovasc Surg. 2016;49(2):99–106. https://doi.org/10.5090/kjtcs.2016.49.2.99. Epub 2016 Apr 5. PubMed PMID: 27066433; PubMed Central PMCID: PMC4825910.

72. Schaible A, Sauer P, Hartwig W, Hackert T, Hinz U, Radeleff B, Büchler MW, Werner J. Radiologic versus endoscopic evaluation of the conduit after esophageal resection: a prospective, blinded, intraindividually controlled diagnostic study. Surg Endosc. 2014;28(7):2078–85. https://doi.org/10.1007/s00464-014-3435-8. Epub 2014 Feb 12. PubMed PMID: 24519029.

73. Shah RD, Luketich JD, Schuchert MJ, Christie NA, Pennathur A, Landreneau RJ, Nason KS. Postesophagectomy chylothorax: incidence, risk factors, and outcomes. Ann Thorac Surg. 2012;93(3):897–903.  https://doi.org/10.1016/j.athoracsur.2011.10.060;  discussion  903–4. Epub 2012 Jan 15. PubMed PMID: 22245587; PubMed Central PMCID: PMC3430511.

74. Dugue L, Sauvanet A, Farges O, Goharin A, Le Mee J, Belghiti J. Output of chyle as an indicator of treatment for chylothorax complicating oesophagectomy. Br J Surg. 1998;85(8):1147–9. PubMed PMID: 9718017.

75. Lott S, Schmieder M, Mayer B, Henne-Bruns D, Knippschild U, Agaimy A, Schwab M, Kramer K. Gastrointestinal stromal tumors of the esophagus: evaluation of a pooled case series regarding clinicopathological features and clinical outcome. Am J Cancer Res. 2014;5(1):333–43. eCollection 2015. PubMed PMID: 25628942; PubMed Central PMCID: PMC4300707.

76. Jiang P, Jiao Z, Han B, Zhang X, Sun X, Su J, Wang C, Gao B. Clinical characteristics and surgical treatment of oesophageal gastrointestinal stromal tumours. Eur J Cardiothorac Surg. 2010;38(2):223–7. https://doi.org/10.1016/j.ejcts.2010.01.040. Epub 2010 Mar 4. PubMed PMID: 20206541.

77. The ESMO/European Sarcoma Network Working Group. Gastrointestinal stromal tumors: ESMO Clinical Practice Guidelines for diagnosis, treatment and follow-up. Ann Oncol. 2012;23(suppl_7):vii49–55. https://doi.org/10.1093/annonc/mds252.

# Figures/Misc.

78. Liete LP, et al. Ineffective esophageal motility (IEM) (the primary finding in patients with nonspecific esophageal motility disorder). Dig Dis Sci. 1997;42(9):1859–65.

79. Posted by K. Eckland. Esophagectomy: modern surgical approaches. Thoracic surgery, 27 Oct. 2014, thoracics.org/2011/11/05/eophagectomy-modern-surgical-approaches/

# Chapter 6
# Gallbladder

**Gian-Paul Vidal and Tomer Davidov**

## Gallstone Disease

### *Epidemiology*

Cholelithiasis is common in the global population with an incidence that is approximately 10% for men and 18% for women [1]. In the United States, 10–20% of the population will have stones, potentially affecting up to 30 million people. However, only about 20% of those people will experience symptoms within 20 years of their diagnosis of cholelithiasis. The annual risk of progression to symptomatic gallstones causing biliary colic, cholecystitis, cholangitis, or pancreatitis is between 1% and 4%; therefore, prophylactic cholecystectomy is not routinely recommended.

With gallstone disease being so common, there are over 750,000 cholecystectomies performed in the United States annually, with the direct and indirect cost totaling over six billion dollars [2]. Cholecystectomy has become the most common elective abdominal surgery in the United States, especially when considering the marked increase in the number of surgeries performed with the advent of the laparoscopic cholecystectomy technique.

Although laparoscopic cholecystectomy is regarded as a relatively benign procedure, it is not risk-free. One report demonstrated a postoperative complication rate of 0.9% and intraoperative common bile duct injuries at 0.1% [3]. Although most complications can be treated conservatively or with endoscopic interventions, it is important to know the indications for surgery to avoid overuse and the options available to treat stone disease nonoperatively, if applicable.

G.-P. Vidal (✉) · T. Davidov
Robert Wood Johnson Medical School, Rutgers University, New Brunswick, NJ, USA
e-mail: vidalgi@rwjms.rutgers.edu; davidoto@rwjms.rutgers.edu

© Springer Nature Switzerland AG 2019
C. Rezac, K. Donohue (eds.), *The Internist's Guide to Minimally Invasive Gastrointestinal Surgery*, Clinical Gastroenterology,
https://doi.org/10.1007/978-3-319-96631-1_6

## Biliary Colic

Biliary colic occurs when there is a temporary obstruction of the cystic duct by a gallstone or sludge. This typically occurs 1–3 h after eating with the subsequent release of cholecystokinin (CCK) stimulating gallbladder contraction. The stones are mobile and not impacted in the neck of the gallbladder, so the pain tends to resolve within 6 h once the obstruction has resolved. Stones that freely pass through the biliary tree do not cause inflammation or symptoms.

The pain in biliary colic is constant, so the term is a misnomer. It is usually localized to the right upper quadrant, but some patients may experience epigastric pain. The pain may radiate to their right shoulder or scapula. Nausea and vomiting are commonly associated symptoms. Patients do not present with jaundice or signs of obstructive hyperbilirubinemia because the common bile duct is patent.

Laboratory testing is usually normal in terms of white blood cell count and hepatic function panel. Transabdominal ultrasonography of the right upper quadrant is the study of choice when biliary colic is suspected and can reveal gallstones, sludge, or polyps. The size of the stones can be measured and it can be noted if they are impacted in the neck of gallbladder. It can also demonstrate if there is gallbladder wall thickening (>3 or 4 mm), pericholecystic fluid, sonographic Murphy's sign (pain in the right upper quadrant with the transducer), and the size of the common bile duct, which if dilated may be suspicious for a common bile duct stone if correlated with an elevated bilirubin and jaundice.

Treatment for symptomatic or minimally symptomatic cholelithiasis is usually nonoperative and includes lifestyle and dietary changes. The decision to operate should be based on a risk-benefit analysis. For patients who have mild symptoms, the risk of complications from gallstones is 1–4% a year, while those with more severe symptoms, the risk increases up to 7% [5]. Patients who are evaluated in the emergency department and present with signs and symptoms classic of biliary colic may safely be discharged home if their pain resolves and they can tolerate food without a recurrence of their pain. The workup should be negative, including normal vital signs, laboratory values, and imaging. On discharge, they are recommended to start a low-fat diet. If the patient has recurrent episodes of biliary colic despite dietary changes, they should be referred to a general surgeon to discuss elective cholecystectomy.

## Acute Cholecystitis

Acute cholecystitis occurs when obstruction of the cystic duct leads to gallbladder inflammation and edema with subserosal hemorrhage. Infection is possible as the obstruction leads to bile stasis, and although bile is considered sterile, gallstones can serve as a nidus for bacteria. Since most biliary infections are gram-negative aerobes, it is thought that bacterial seeding occurs upward from the duodenum through the biliary tree. Acute cholecystitis, if left untreated, can progress to acute gangrenous cholecystitis. At this stage, the gallbladder may perforate leading to bile peritonitis. If there is a superimposed infection with gas-forming organisms, it is termed acute emphysematous cholecystitis.

Patients suffering from acute cholecystitis typically present with unrelenting right upper quadrant pain and tenderness to palpation on examination with a positive Murphy's sign (cessation of deep inspiration while pressure is applied under the right costal margin). They may also present with fevers, chills, nausea, and vomiting.

The diagnosis of acute cholecystitis can be aided with laboratory testing and imaging. Patients with suspected acute cholecystitis may have a leukocytosis. Hyperbilirubinemia, as well as an elevation of alkaline phosphatase and transaminases, should raise suspicion for choledocholithiasis and even cholangitis if associated with fever and jaundice. Ultrasonography may reveal a distended gallbladder with wall thickening and pericholecystic fluid (Fig. 6.1a, b). A stone impacted in the neck of the gallbladder is commonly seen. A CT scan may show similar changes as the ultrasound, and it can also demonstrate emphysematous changes. A hepatic iminodiacetic acid scan (HIDA) can demonstrate if the cystic duct is obstructed.

The treatment for acute cholecystitis is cholecystectomy, with the laparoscopic approach being the gold standard. The timing of when to operate was a topic of debate, but studies have shown that early laparoscopic cholecystectomy (within a week of symptoms) compared to delayed cholecystectomy (after nonoperative treatment with antibiotics and a 6-week interval) can be performed with improved morbidity, a decrease in length of stay, and total hospital cost, with a similar conversion rate to open cholecystectomy [4]. Additionally, studies showed that a significant number of patients treated nonoperatively would return to the emergency department with a recurrent episode of cholecystitis or unremitting symptoms prior to their scheduled interval laparoscopic cholecystectomy.

A patient with suspected acute cholecystitis should be evaluated by a general surgeon. If the diagnosis is made, the patient should be admitted to the surgical

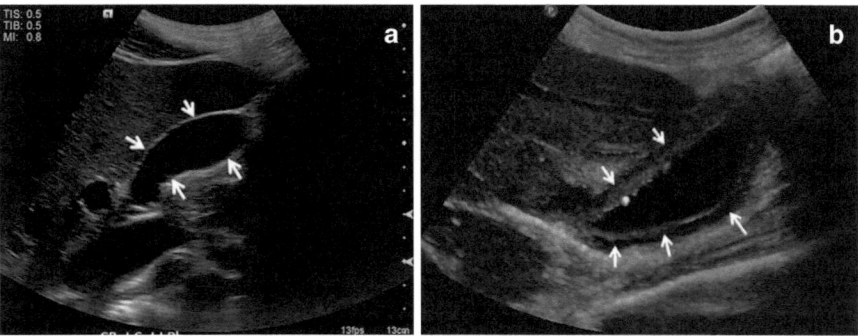

**Fig. 6.1 a** RUQ ultrasound of a normal thin-walled gallbladder. **b** RUQ ultrasound showing a thickened, edematous gallbladder wall consistent with acute cholecystitis. (Used with permission. de Virgilio [8])

service, made nothing per os, started on intravenous fluids and broad-spectrum antibiotics, and given parenteral pain medication and antiemetics to keep the patient comfortable while they await their cholecystectomy.

## Chronic Cholecystitis

Chronic cholecystitis occurs when recurrent episodes of biliary colic and partial cystic duct obstruction eventually lead to fibrosis of the gallbladder neck and the cystic duct. Patients present with similar symptoms as biliary colic, although their pain may occur much more frequently and may no longer be associated with food. They may also present with bloating, nausea, and vomiting.

Laboratory findings may be normal, and ultrasonography may reveal stones and gallbladder wall thickening. The treatment is cholecystectomy.

## Choledocholithiasis

Choledocholithiasis occurs when there is a stone in the common bile duct. The stones most commonly arise in the gallbladder (secondary stones) but, rarely, may arise in the bile duct itself (primary stones). Many common bile duct stones are silent, but when they are symptomatic, they can present along a spectrum of syndromes ranging from biliary colic to acute cholangitis. Patients may present with elevated alkaline phosphatase and hyperbilirubinemia along the symptomatology of obstructive jaundice, icterus, dark colored urine, and acholic stools.

Ultrasonography may show choledocholithiasis or an abnormally dilated common bile duct. Even if stones are not visualized, a patient presenting with cholelithiasis, a dilated common bile duct, and an elevated bilirubin should be evaluated for choledocholithiasis with further imaging. Magnetic resonance cholangiopancreatography (MRCP) is very sensitive (>90%) and specific (~100%) for evaluating choledocholithiasis. Since it is less invasive than endoscopic retrograde cholangiopancreatography (ERCP), many physicians and gastroenterologists will start with MRCP prior to deciding to utilize ERCP. Endoscopic ultrasound (EUS) is more accurate than MRCP for the detection of bile duct stones and does not carry the risk of iatrogenic pancreatitis, but it is only a diagnostic tool and is not therapeutic like ERCP.

ERCP is highly sensitive and specific for choledocholithiasis and can be therapeutic with its ability to clear out the stones. During the procedure, the gastroenterologist performs a cholangiogram in order to visualize the biliary anatomy and detect any filling defects within the ducts, presumably stones. They may perform a sphincterotomy and extract the stones. A temporary stent may be left. Important risks of ERCP include pancreatitis, intestinal perforation, and recurrence of choledocholithiasis.

Intraoperatively, a patient can undergo a laparoscopic cholangiogram to identify choledocholithiasis. Based on the surgeon's experience, they may be able to extract the stones by either laparoscopic or open common bile duct exploration. With the frequent use of laparoscopic and endoscopic techniques, open duct exploration is less common. Another common method is for the patient to undergo a postoperative ERCP to remove any stones identified in the operating room.

In patients with choledocholithiasis who are managed by ERCP and sphincterotomy alone, almost half will have a recurrence; therefore, it is recommended that the patient undergoes a laparoscopic cholecystectomy during the same admission. However, in patients older than 70 years of age, the rate of recurrence is about 15%, so a cholecystectomy may be selectively offered.

After a cholecystectomy, a patient may present with choledocholithiasis. If this occurs within 2 years of surgery, the stones are thought to be secondary and are termed *retained*. If it occurs after 2 years, then they are *recurrent* primary common bile duct stones.

## Cholangitis

Cholangitis refers to a life-threatening ascending infection of the biliary tree caused by an acute biliary obstruction. There should be a high degree of suspicion in a patient who presents with right upper quadrant tenderness, jaundice, and fevers—commonly known as *Charcot's triad*. If left untreated, a patient can progress and display *Reynold's pentad*, which includes hypotension and altered mental status suggestive of shock.

Treatment of cholangitis includes intravenous broad-spectrum antibiotics and fluid resuscitation and emergent decompression of the biliary tree either by percutaneous transhepatic cholangiography (PTC) or ERCP. It is not advised for the patient to undergo surgery as a first-line treatment. In some centers, it is possible to perform an intraoperative ERCP at the time of laparoscopic cholecystectomy, a procedure known as "laparoendoscopic rendezvous."

## Gallstone Ileus

Gallstone ileus is a misnomer as it is in fact a small bowel obstruction caused by the erosion of a very large gallstone from the gallbladder into the duodenum creating a cholecystoduodenal fistula. The stone then travels through the gastrointestinal tract and becomes lodged in the ileocecal valve—the narrowest portion of the tract. Patients typically present with the signs and symptoms of a small bowel obstruction including abdominal pain, nausea, vomiting, and changes in bowel habits. Diagnosis can be made with imaging such as a CT scan showing pneumobilia and a large stone in the small intestine (Fig. 6.2). Since these patients tend to be older and very sick,

**Fig. 6.2** Gallstone ileus
showing large stone (red
arrow) and pneumobilia
(yellow arrow). (Used
with permission. Liau
et al. [9])

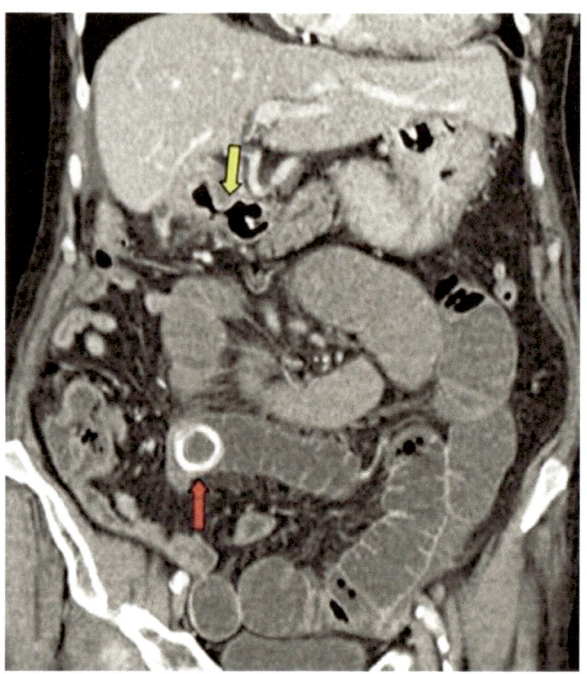

the primary goal of an operation is to relieve the obstruction by creating an enterotomy on the healthy bowel proximal to the stone and then milking it out. After
ensuring there are no more stones in the small intestine, the enterotomy is closed.
There may be very dense adhesions in the right upper quadrant, so cholecystectomy
and fistula closure are usually postponed until the patient has improved, and the
operation is deemed safe given a patient's comorbidities.

## Gallstone Pancreatitis

Gallstone pancreatitis is another complication caused by cholelithiasis. Patients
who present with pancreatitis should be treated medically. Surgical consultation
should be requested for a planned cholecystectomy prior to discharge once the pancreatitis has resolved.

# Biliary Dysfunction

## Biliary Dyskinesia

Biliary dyskinesia is a motility disorder of the gallbladder. It typically presents with
symptoms classic of calculous biliary disease, but there is no evidence of stones on

imaging. During workup, the patient should have other causes of right upper quadrant pain ruled out by imaging and upper endoscopy. If the workup remains negative and the patient's symptoms appear highly suggestive of biliary colic, a CCK-stimulated HIDA scan may be obtained to check for gallbladder dysfunction. If the scan shows an ejection fraction less than 35%, it is diagnostic for biliary dyskinesia. There is no effective medical treatment for dyskinesia, so laparoscopic cholecystectomy is the gold standard. It has been proven to be effective for 85% of patients [5]. If patients continue to have symptoms postoperatively, further evaluation with a gastroenterologist is indicated.

## Sphincter of Oddi Dysfunction (SOD)

The sphincter of Oddi is the muscular sphincter found at the ampulla of Vater or the hepatopancreatic ampulla. Its primary functions are to control of the flow of biliary and digestive juices into the second portion of the duodenum, divert bile into the gallbladder, and prevent reflux of bile and intestinal content into the pancreatic duct. Abnormalities in the anatomy or function of the sphincter can lead to biliary pain. Dysfunction of the sphincter can be from abnormal spasms of the muscle or secondary to fibrosis of the sphincter due to trauma, pancreatitis, the passage of gallstones, or congenital anomalies.

Patients with SOD present with right upper quadrant or upper abdominal pain that is constant and lasts for at least 30 min. Patients may also present with recurrent episodes of pancreatitis. SOD should be suspected if a patient presents with upper abdominal pain, abnormal hepatopancreatic enzyme levels, and a common bile duct size greater than 12 mm on ultrasound. The diagnosis can be confirmed with manometry if the basal sphincter pressure is greater than 40 mmHg. However, this is a highly sophisticated technique only available at specialized gastroenterology centers.

Treatment for SOD is endoscopic sphincterotomy, which has been effective in 60–90% of patients [5].

## Cholecystectomy

### Laparoscopic Cholecystectomy

Since the 1990s, with the advent of laparoscopy surgery, cholecystectomies can be performed safely for biliary colic and for acute and chronic cholecystitis. Laparoscopy surgery is associated with decreased length of stay, decreased complications, and less postoperative pain. However, it has been associated with an increase in common bile duct injuries that may require extensive repair and reconstruction.

During the operation, the patient is placed in a supine position with both arms extended outward to the side. Perioperative antibiotics are administered if there is a concern for cholecystitis. Sequential compression devices are placed on both legs unless there is a contraindication, and venous thromboembolism prophylaxis may be given at the surgeon's discretion. The patient then undergoes general endotracheal anesthesia and is prepped and draped in a sterile fashion. An orogastric tube may be inserted to decompress the stomach and improve visualization. A Foley catheter may be inserted.

There are a variety of methods to enter the abdomen, but the location of the incisions and laparoscopic ports tends to be standard. There are four incisions in total: one around the umbilicus, one located subxiphoid, and two on the patient's right lateral side. The periumbilical incision tends to be the largest incision at 10–12 mm, since this is where the specimen will be extracted. The remaining incisions are usually 5 mm. The periumbilical incision is created first in order to insert the laparoscope (camera) and the remaining ports under direct visual guidance.

Using graspers and blunt dissectors, the gallbladder is retracted and freed from peritoneal adhesions to expose the cystic duct and the cystic artery. Many surgeons urge achieving this critical view of safety before transecting any structures to avoid common bile duct injuries (Fig. 6.3). This generally entails clearing the hepatocystic triangle of any fibrous tissue and visualizing only two structures directly entering the gallbladder—presumably the cystic duct and artery. The liver bed should be seen in the space between these two structures.

At times, it may be necessary to perform an intraoperative cholangiogram to delineate the biliary anatomy as well as to determine whether there are any common bile duct stones. In order to do so, the presumed cystic duct is partially transected, and a catheter is inserted and secured with a clip. Contrast is injected into the duct and visualized using fluoroscopy. This can help the surgeon identify the cystic duct, common bile duct, and even choledocholithiasis. If there are stones present, the surgeon may attempt to flush them with the aid of glucagon as it relaxes the sphincter of Oddi.

If the surgeon is confident the cystic duct and cystic artery have been identified, then the structures are doubly clipped on the patient's side and singly clipped on the specimen side before being transected with scissors. Once they are divided, the gallbladder is freed from the liver bed using electrocautery. The gallbladder is then placed in a bag and extracted through the umbilical incision along with the trocar.

**Fig. 6.3** The critical view showing the cystic duct, cystic artery, and the liver bed. (Used with permission. Halverson [10])

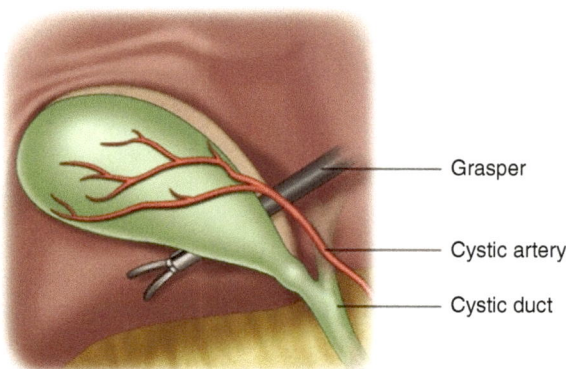

Grasper

Cystic artery

Cystic duct

The periumbilical trocar and laparoscope are reinserted. The gallbladder fossa is inspected for hemostasis, and the clips on the stumps of the cystic artery and cystic duct are confirmed to be in proper place. The field can be irrigated if there was spillage of bile, stones, or pus. It is always important to note the spillage of stones, especially if they have not been retrieved, because they carry a risk of infection and complications later on. Once everything is satisfactory, the trocars are removed under direct visualization, and the abdomen is de-sufflated. A drain may be placed if there is a concern for potential bile leak. The fascia of the periumbilical incision is closed to prevent a port-site hernia since the defect is larger than 1 cm. The skin of all the incisions is usually approximated with a dissolvable subcuticular suture. Skin glue or a sterile gauze dressing is then applied to the incisions.

The operation can take anywhere from 30 min to 3–4 h depending on the severity of inflammation of the gallbladder. Patients can generally go home the same day or the following morning. Antibiotics postoperatively are at the discretion of the surgeon based on intraoperative findings, but usually 24 h of perioperative antibiotics is sufficient. Patients are instructed to restrict any lifting to 15–20 lbs. for 6 weeks to prevent an incisional hernia, especially at the umbilicus. Patients tend to return to work several days later. Although they do not have any dietary restrictions with the gallbladder removed, patients may experience loose stools or diarrhea with fatty meals initially, but it is self-limited.

In cases with severe inflammation from cholecystitis, the gallbladder may not be removed safely, laparoscopically or open. In these circumstances, a partial cholecystectomy may be performed. This may proceed in two ways. One method is to divide the gallbladder and leave behind the posterior wall adhered to the liver bed (Fig. 6.4a). The remnant gallbladder wall is cauterized to prevent a bile leak, and the internal opening of the cystic duct is over sewn (Fig. 6.4b, c). In these cases, and others where there is concern for a potential bile leak, a drain is placed.

The second method is to transect the gallbladder at the level of the infundibulum with a stapler if it is not possible to safely dissect out and identify the cystic artery and cystic duct (Fig. 6.5).

## Single-Port Laparoscopic Cholecystectomy

It is possible to perform a laparoscopic cholecystectomy using a single 2 cm periumbilical incision and a specialized trocar that accommodates the camera and instruments. Studies have shown this technique has a greater learning curve than traditional laparoscopy, but experienced surgeons may have decreased operative times compared to a standard multi-port approach. In addition, the surgeon always has the capability to insert additional trocars in order to aid with retraction. There is also an improvement in cosmesis as the patient will have a single scar.

Single-port cholecystectomy is safe and comparable with the standard approach in terms of hospital length of stay; however, an increase in incisional hernias has been reported after single-port surgeries.

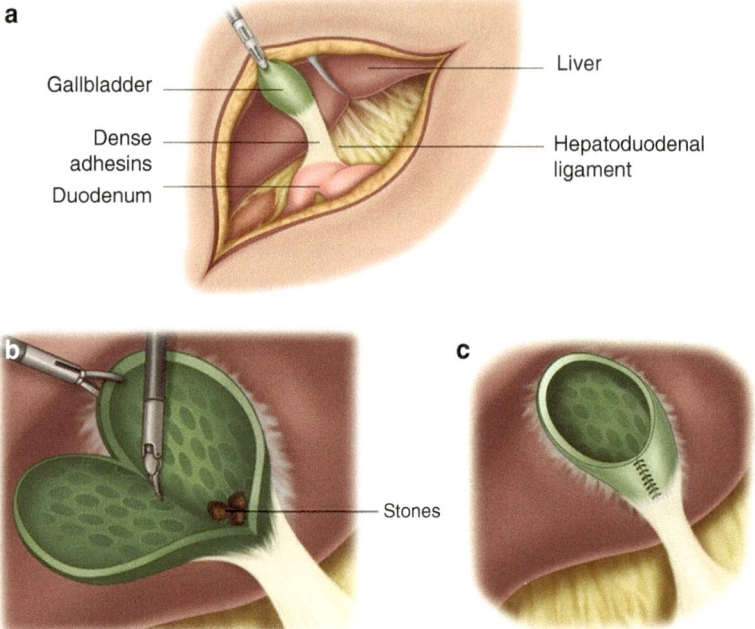

**Fig. 6.4** **a** Dense adhesions impair ability to identify cystic structures and increase risk of biliary injuries. **b** The gallbladder is divided with electrocautery, leaving the posterior wall on the liver bed. **c** The remnant wall is cauterized, and the infundibulum sutured closed. (Used with permission. Halverson [10])

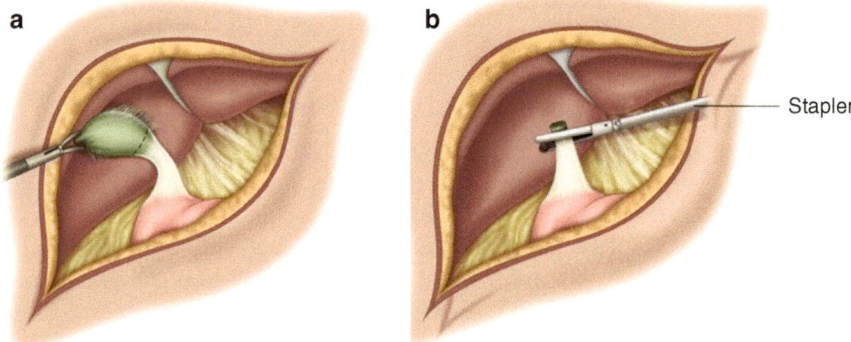

**Fig. 6.5** **a** Full mobilization of the fundus of the gallbladder. **b** Stapled amputation of gallbladder. (Used with permission. Halverson [10])

# da Vinci *Robotic-Assisted Cholecystectomy*

Robotic-assisted surgeries have provided surgeons with many benefits during an operation. They allow for a much more ergonomic, seated position, provide a three-dimensional operative view, and increase the surgeon's dexterity with articulated instruments.

As with laparoscopy, it is possible to perform the operation using a multi-port or single-port approach with the robot. Robotic cholecystectomies are safe to perform and have the added benefit of using fluorescent imaging to perform intraoperative cholangiograms to visualize difficult biliary anatomy. However, robotic cholecystectomies may be associated with longer operating room times in order to dock the machine, as well as higher hospital costs. Figure 6.6 demonstrates a typical setup for robotic- assisted surgery as well as the larger port for single-site operations.

## *Open Cholecystectomy*

Open cholecystectomy is the traditional approach to removing the gallbladder. It involves a large right oblique incision that runs parallel to the costal margin. Conversion to open cholecystectomy is most commonly performed in order to avoid injuring the common bile duct because of unclear biliary anatomy. Although the conversion rate is as low as 1% [6], all patients should be consented and prepared for it. Other reasons for conversion include uncontrolled bleeding, the need for common bile duct exploration, and suspected common bile duct injury. After an open procedure, most patients will stay in the hospital for a couple of days for adequate pain control. They have the same weight lifting and exercising restrictions as the laparoscopic approach.

## *Common Bile Duct Exploration*

Depending on surgical expertise, common bile duct exploration may be performed open or laparoscopically. Nowadays, many surgeons will elect to have the patient undergo postoperative ERCP if there is suspicion for choledocholithiasis.

## Postcholecystectomy Considerations

Postcholecystectomy syndrome is used to describe when a patient experiences a recurrence of their biliary symptoms after cholecystectomy. It can occur in 10–15%

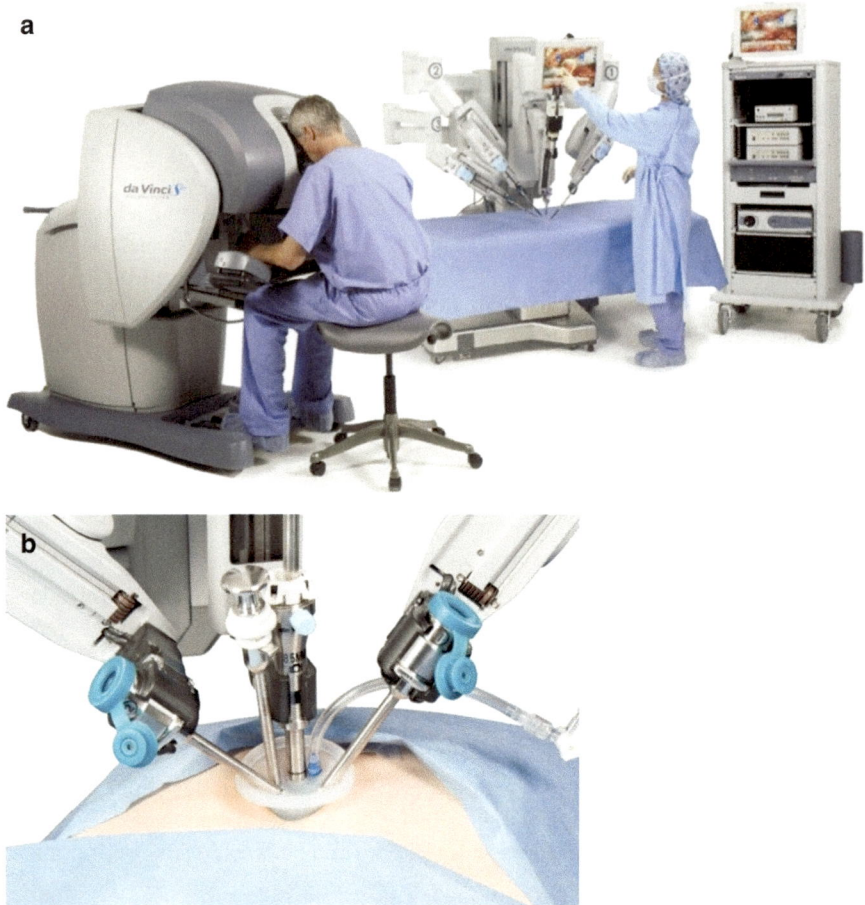

**Fig. 6.6** **a** Full view of a *da Vinci S HD* system. **b** Single-Site™ final docked position. (© 2018 Intuitive Surgical, Inc.)

of patients after surgery. Patients experience abdominal pain, nausea, vomiting, dyspepsia, and diarrhea. One common thought is that there is an increase in the amount of bile that enters the intestines since the gallbladder no longer acts a reservoir. The diagnosis should be one of exclusion.

## Bile Leak

A bile leak can occur from an injury to the bile duct, a cystic duct stump leak, or from the ducts of Lushka (small accessory ducts that drain directly into the gallbladder from the liver). Patients may present with new, worsening abdominal pain, nausea, vomiting, a leukocytosis, and/or transaminitis.

Ultrasonography or CT imaging can show the presence of a biloma or abscess. The presence of an active leak can be made with a HIDA scan or an ERCP cholangiogram. ERCP can be therapeutic with its ability to perform a sphincterotomy and place a stent. This will redirect the flow of bile through the path of least resistance allowing the leak to heal. The biloma or abscess should then be drained percutaneously with the help of interventional radiologists.

Cystic stump leaks are rare, occurring after less than 1% of laparoscopic cholecystectomies [7]. They may occur if the clips on the cystic duct are displaced. This may be due to necrosis of the cystic duct stump or from back pressure of bile from stones in the common bile duct.

Leaks from the ducts of Lushka may also present in a similar form and are treated the same.

## Bile Duct Injury

If a bile duct injury is recognized intraoperatively during a laparoscopic cholecystectomy, conversion to an operation is necessary in order to assess the degree of injury and formulate a plan. The goal is to preserve as much of the duct as possible and create a tension-free repair, either primarily over a T-tube or via a biliary-enteric reconstruction (e.g., hepaticojejunostomy, choledochojejunostomy). If the surgeon does not have the expertise, it is acceptable to leave a drain in order to control the bile leak and transfer the patient to a hepatobiliary specialist.

In patients in whom the injury is not diagnosed immediately, they may present with new onset pain, jaundice, elevated alkaline phosphate and bilirubin levels, and a bile leak. The bile leak may be in the form of a biloma or as bilious drainage from the incisions.

A CT scan may reveal a sterile biloma or abscess that would require percutaneous drainage. An ERCP or percutaneous transhepatic cholangiogram (PTC) is necessary to delineate the biliary anatomy in order to guide planning for operative repair. During a PTC, transhepatic drainage catheters may be placed to help control drainage and assist in operative dissection.

## Spilled Gallstones

During laparoscopic surgery, it is not uncommon for the gallbladder to be inadvertently opened and for stones to be spilled. The surgeon should make an effort to irrigate the field and retrieve as many stones as possible. The stones can serve as a nidus for infection and cause complications in the long term such as abscess formation, bowel obstructions, and fistulas.

# References

1. Shaffer EA. Epidemiology of gallbladder stone disease. Best Pract Res Clin Gastroenterol. 2006;20(5):981–96.
2. Stinton LM, Shaffer EA. Epidemiology of gallbladder disease: cholelithiasis and cancer. Gut Liver. 2012;6(2):172–87.
3. Duca S, Bālā O, Al-Hajjar N, Lancu C, Puia IC, Munteanu D, Graur F. Laparoscopic cholecystectomy: incidents and complications: a retrospective analysis of 9542 consecutive laparoscopic operations. HPB. 2003;5(3):152–8.
4. Gutt CN, Encke J, Köninger J, Harnoss JC, Weigand K, Kipfmüller K, et al. Acute cholecystitis: early versus delayed cholecystectomy, a multicenter randomized trial. Ann Surg. 2013;3:385–93.
5. Jackson PG, Evans S. Biliary system. In: Townsend CM, Beauchamp D, Evers M, Mattox K, editors. Sabiston textbook of surgery: the biological basis of modern surgical practice. 19th ed. Philadelphia: Elsevier Saunders; 2012. p. 1485–500.
6. Bingener-Casey J, Richards ML, Strodel WE, Schwesinger WH, Sirinek KR. Reasons for conversion from laparoscopic to open cholecystectomy: a 10-year review. J Gastrointestinal Surgery. 2002;6(6):800–5.
7. Unger WS, Glick GL, Landeros M. Cystic duct leak after laparoscopic cholecystectomy, a multi-national study. Surg Endosc. 1996;10(12):1189–93.
8. de Virgilio C, et al. Surgery: a case based clinical review. New York: Springer; 2015.
9. Liau SS, et al. A case of gallstone-induced small bowel necrosis masquerading as clinical appendicitis. Clin J Gastroenterol. 2009;2:239.
10. Halverson AL. Advanced surgical techniques for rural surgeons. New York: Springer; 2015.

# Chapter 7
# Minimally Invasive Liver Surgery

Ioannis Konstantinidis and Laleh Melstrom

## Introduction

Minimally invasive surgery is associated with faster recovery and equivalent oncologic outcomes compared to open surgery for resections involving a variety of
organs, including the colon [1], esophagus [2], and stomach [3]. From the time of
the first description of a laparoscopic nonanatomic liver resection for focal nodular
hyperplasia in 1992 [4], its expansion has been tremendous, with 2804 cases
reported in 2009 and more than 9000 cases reported in 2016 [5, 6]. Similar to other
organs, minimally invasive liver surgery appears to be associated with improved
short-term outcomes (smaller incisions, decreased blood loss, shorter hospitalization, fewer complications) and equivalent oncologic outcomes when performed for
cancer [5–8].

Patient selection is paramount as minimally invasive liver surgery entails unique
challenges. For instance, it cannot be utilized in patients unable to tolerate pneumoperitoneum, and it is technically more challenging in the presence of extensive
adhesions. In addition, minimally invasive approaches entail a learning curve,
whereas major bleeding might be difficult to control and require conversion to open
surgery. Procedure-specific risks such as gas embolism appear to be an exceedingly
rare phenomenon [5, 6].

The introduction of robotic technology for minimally invasive liver procedures is
an attempt to overcome some of the limitations of conventional laparoscopy. The
benefits of robotic-assisted surgery can be visual (increased magnification, three-
dimensional view, improved depth of perception) and also ergonomic/technical
(seven ranges of motion versus four of laparoscopy, motion scaling of the robot,

I. Konstantinidis · L. Melstrom (✉)
Department of Surgery, City of Hope Medical Center, Duarte, CA, USA
e-mail: ikonstantinidis@coh.org; lmelstrom@coh.org

© Springer Nature Switzerland AG 2019                                                    93
C. Rezac, K. Donohue (eds.), *The Internist's Guide to Minimally Invasive
Gastrointestinal Surgery*, Clinical Gastroenterology,
https://doi.org/10.1007/978-3-319-96631-1_7

tremor filtration, articulating instruments), which render the robot beneficial for precise surgical dissection and fine suturing, even in narrow operative fields [9]. These features make the robotic platform particularly attractive for liver surgery and advantageous for procedures such as portal lymphadenectomy, biliary reconstruction, and resection of posterior/superior liver segments [10]. A recent review of robotic oncologic surgery showed that robotic surgery is widely used for a variety of operations and for several procedures, with evidence that robotics offer short-term benefits with comparable safety profiles and oncologic outcomes to open surgery [11]. However, robotic technology is not without drawbacks. The cost is significantly higher, there is need for specialized training (surgeon, skilled bedside assistant and nurses), and some technical issues common to laparoscopy remain unsolved, such as the absence of haptic feedback. Thus, new technologies are being investigated and are expected to address some of these limitations.

## From Introduction to Adoption of Minimally Invasive Liver Surgery

The introduction of minimally invasive liver surgery into routine surgical practice created the need of a formal framework to examine its indications and the associated risks and benefits. There have been already two international consensus conferences on minimally invasive liver surgery [12, 13]. The first conference set the terminology and an initial approach to the indications of laparoscopic liver surgery, and the second investigated the accumulated evidence on the use of minimally invasive liver surgery, including robotic surgery, for minor and major hepatic resections [12]. Three techniques were described during the first meeting: pure laparoscopy, where the entire operation is performed laparoscopically; the hand-assisted approach with utilization of a hand port; and the hybrid method, where the resection is performed through a minilaparotomy incision. The indications for minimally invasive liver surgery were solitary lesions of less than 5 cm in size, at the peripheral liver segments 2–6. Laparoscopic left lateral sectionectomy was considered standard practice, whereas major liver resections were appropriate only for experienced surgeons in advanced laparoscopy.

Correlating with these recommendations, a summary of the reported worldwide laparoscopic liver experience from over 2800 surgeries published during the same year revealed that 65% of the resections were minor (45% wedge resections or segmentectomies), 16% were lobectomies, and 50% were performed for malignancy, with conversion rates at 4%. The majority of the liver procedures performed were laparoscopies (75%), 17% were hand-assisted operations, and 2% were hybrid procedures, with perioperative morbidity and mortality of 11% and 0.3%, respectively [6].

Almost 6 years later, a second international conference examined the interim worldwide accumulated experience. Even though the level of existing evidence was deemed to be too weak to provide strong recommendations, minor liver resections were considered standard practice, whereas major hepatectomies were still considered being in an exploratory phase. No specific recommendations were made for robotic surgery with the current literature, suggesting no inferior outcomes to other techniques [13].

These trends are being reflected in recent studies. In a recent report utilizing the liver module of the American College of Surgeons National Surgical Quality Improvement Program and data from 2448 patients, laparoscopic procedures consisted only 21.4% of the cases, whereas robotic surgery constituted 1.1%. The percentages for major hepatectomies were even lower, with 11.7% performed laparoscopically and 0.6% robotically [14]. A recent review of more than 9000 laparoscopic liver resections showed that 65% were performed for malignancy and illustrated both the safety of laparoscopic liver surgery (mortality rate was very low 0.4%) and its improved postoperative outcome for minor and major hepatectomies, whereas the numbers of major and complex resections are increasing but remain mostly limited to expert centers [5]. At the same time, in Europe, a consensus statement on the use of robotics in general surgery supported that robotic assistance might facilitate complex biliary surgery, especially bilioenteric bypass. Moreover, robotic hepatectomy has comparable clinical outcomes to laparoscopic hepatectomy, and the use of robotic assistance may increase the rate of minimally invasive major hepatic resections [15].

## Comparative Studies

Minimally invasive liver surgery has theoretical advantages over open liver surgery, including the magnified view and the presence of pneumoperitoneum, which reduces bleeding from the low-pressure hepatic veins [16]. There are no published randomized controlled trials comparing open to minimally invasive liver surgery or laparoscopic to robotic liver surgery. However, there are many ongoing trials in Europe on laparoscopic versus open liver surgery for colorectal cancer liver metastases, such as the Netherlands, Norway, and Spain trials (ClinicalTrials.gov identifiers: NCT01441856, NCT01516710, NCT02727179, respectively) and similarly in China and Japan on hepatocellular cancer (ClinicalTrials.gov identifiers: NCT01768741 and NCT00606385, respectively), which are expected to provide further evidence on the advantages of laparoscopic liver surgery.

Overall, the existing evidence attests to superior postoperative outcomes for minimally invasive over open liver surgery and to equivalent outcomes between laparoscopic and robotic liver surgery. Table 7.1 summarizes some important comparative studies. A meta-analysis of open versus laparoscopic surgery for hepatocellular cancer showed that the laparoscopic approach was associated with less blood loss, fewer complications, and shorter hospital stay with no differences in surgical margins [17]. Importantly, the long-term oncologic outcome is not compromised. A meta-analysis of studies on laparoscopic versus open liver resection focusing on long-term outcomes and analyzing separately hepatocellular cancer and colorectal liver metastases patients found no differences in the 1-, 3-, or 5-year survival rates [18]. Two recently published multi-institutional reports from Japan (Table 7.1), utilizing data from over 4700 patients who underwent surgery for colorectal cancer

**Table 7.1** Selected comparative studies on minimally invasive liver resections

| Comparison | Year/type | N | Operative outcome | Oncologic outcome | Author conclusions | Study |
|---|---|---|---|---|---|---|
| LLR vs. OLR | Multi-institutional PSM analysis | CRCLM:<br>LLR: 171<br>OLR: 342<br>HCC:<br>LLR: 387<br>OLR: 387 | LLR:<br>Less EBL<br>Shorter hospital stay<br>Similar MM (less morbidity in HCC study) | Similar R0<br>RFS<br>DSS | LLR:<br>Lower blood loss<br>Shorter hospital stay<br>Equivalent survival<br>Less complications in HCC population | [8, 19] |
| LLR vs. OLR | 2016/meta-analysis | 2900 | LLR:<br>Less EBL<br>Shorter hospital stay<br>Morbidity | Similar R0 | LLR:<br>May offer improved short-term outcomes | [5] |
| RLR vs. OLR | Single institution PSM analysis | RLR: 183<br>OLR: 275 | RLR:<br>Less EBL<br>Shorter hospital stay<br>Similar MM | Similar R0<br>RFS<br>DSS | RLR:<br>Less postoperative pain and shorter stay | [30] |
| RLR vs. LLR | 2016/meta-analysis | RLR: 254<br>LRL: 522 | Similar EBL<br>Similar hospital stay<br>Similar morbidity | Similar R0 | Similar safety<br>Feasibility<br>Effectiveness | [20] |

Notes: *CRCLM* colorectal cancer liver metastases, *DSS* disease-specific survival, *EBL* estimated blood loss, *HCC* hepatocellular cancer, *LLR* laparoscopic liver resection, *MM* morbidity and mortality, *NA* not applicable, *OLR* open liver resection, *PSM* propensity score matching, *R0* margin-negative resections, *RFS* recurrence-free survival, *RLR* robotic liver resection liver metastases and hepatocellular cancer and matching open and laparoscopic groups with propensity score matching, confirmed the improved short-term outcome and equivalent long-term outcome associated with laparoscopic liver resection [8, 19]. In a recent review of more than 9000 laparoscopic liver resections and meta-analysis, laparoscopic liver surgery was found to have an improved postoperative outcome both for minor and major hepatectomies (Table 7.1).

Comparing laparoscopic to robotic liver surgery shows similar outcomes. A meta-analysis of robotic versus laparoscopic hepatectomy showed evidence of similar safety and effectiveness with higher cost for the robotic hepatectomies [20] (Table 7.1). Tsung et al. [21] in a matched comparison of laparoscopic and robotic liver resections reported similar estimated blood loss, conversion rates, complications, and length of stay with the outcomes of robotic surgery improving with accumulated experience. A multi-institutional Italian study similarly found similar perioperative outcomes for major hepatectomies between the robotic and laparoscopic approach [22]. Wu et al. in a study from Taiwan found conversion to open, morbidity, and mortality rates comparable with greater operative time and blood loss for the robotic group [23]. The worldwide experienced surgery centers from the USA, Europe, and Asia concur about their equivalent results of laparoscopic and robotic liver surgery.

## Challenges and Future Directions

It is important to realize that minimally invasive liver surgery comes with a steep learning curve, and there is definitely selection bias in patients subjected to minimally invasive surgery, even in matched cohorts. The presence of a learning curve is well described for both laparoscopic and robotic-assisted liver surgery. With accumulating experience by the surgeon and health personnel, the conversion rates, operative times, and estimated blood loss decrease, and morbidity improves. The number of cases to achieve improved outcomes might be as high as 60 for laparoscopic major hepatectomy [24] and more than 50 for robotic major hepatectomy [25]. Ways to facilitate learning and shorten the learning curve are being investigated. For example, the use of the robotic dual console is a teaching tool that could help accelerate proficiency [26]. In addition, various teaching curricula are currently being developed and tested, such as the Fundamentals of Robotic Surgery (FRS) (http://FRsurgery.org).

Equally important is to realize that minimally invasive and open liver surgery should not be viewed as competitive approaches. Conversion to a hybrid procedure may be needed when patient safety renders it, and it can maintain the benefits of minimally invasive liver surgery without compromising its safety.

One of the great benefits of minimally invasive surgery, especially robotic surgery, is the relatively ease of incorporation of new technologies targeting better visualization of anatomical structures or improved ergonomics. For example, indocyanine green (ICG) is a nontoxic fluorophore that appears green when stimulated by near-infrared light. It is FDA-approved, and following IV injection, it accumulates in the liver and is secreted in the bile within 45–60 min. Intraoperative indocyanine green fluorescence imaging (IGFI) facilitates recognition of vascular and biliary anatomy and can assist in identifying liver tumors as well as the boundaries of liver segments, aiming at increasing the surgical accuracy. Fusion IGFI can achieve tridimensional (3D) parenchymal demarcation clearer than the conventional demarcation technique [27]. A concerning ergonomical obstacle, the absence of haptic feedback is a widely accepted limitation of robotic surgery. New robotic surgical systems that promise to improve/allow/simulate haptic feedback are under development or already being tested in animal models and are expected to overcome this weakness and create conditions of less tissue damage [28].

Laparoscopic surgery continues to evolve as well. One of the major limitations of conventional laparoscopy is the lack of depth perception. This has been corrected with the introduction of 3D imaging in laparoscopic surgery. 3D visualization in laparoscopic liver surgery is now feasible and may be associated with a decrease in the operative time [29]. Minimally invasive surgery is going through its evolution phase, and exciting new opportunities are on the rise.

**Acknowledgment** We would like to thank Indra Mahajan PhD for her critical editorial review of this manuscript.

# References

1. Clinical outcomes of Surgical Therapy Study Group, Nelsoh H, Sargent DJ, Wileand HS, Fleshman J, Anvari M, Stryker SJ, Beart RW Jr, Hwllinger M, Flanagan R Jr, Peters W, Ota D. A comparison of laparoscopically assisted and open colectomy for colon cancer. N Engl J Med. 2004;350(20):2050–9. Epub 2004/05/14. eng.
2. Biere SS, Cuesta MA, van der Peet DL. Minimally invasive versus open esophagectomy for cancer: a systematic review and meta-analysis. Minerva Chir. 2009;64(2):121–33. Epub 2009/04/15. eng.
3. Vinuela EF, Gonen M, Brennan MF, Coit DG, Strong VE. Laparoscopic versus open distal gastrectomy for gastric cancer: a meta-analysis of randomized controlled trials and high-quality nonrandomized studies. Ann Surg. 2012;255(3):446–56. Epub 2012/02/15. eng.
4. Gagner MRM, Dubuc J. Laparoscopic partial hepatectomy for liver tumor (abstract). Surg Endosc. 1992;6(99):99.
5. Ciria R, Cherqui D, Geller DA, Briceno J, Wakabayashi G. Comparative Short-term Benefits of Laparoscopic Liver Resection: 9000 Cases and Climbing. Ann Surg. 2016;263(4):761–77. Epub 2015/12/25. eng.
6. Nguyen KT, Gamblin TC, Geller DA. World review of laparoscopic liver resection-2,804 patients. Ann Surg. 2009;250(5):831–41.
7. Martin RC, Scoggins CR, McMasters KM. Laparoscopic hepatic lobectomy: advantages of a minimally invasive approach. J Am Coll Surg. 2010;210(5):627–34, 34–6.
8. Beppu T, Wakabayashi G, Hasegawa K, Gotohda N, Mizuguchi T, Takahashi Y, et al. Long-term and perioperative outcomes of laparoscopic versus open liver resection for colorectal liver metastases with propensity score matching: a multi-institutional Japanese study. J Hepatobiliary Pancreat Sci. 2015;22(10):711–20.
9. Ji WB, Wang HG, Zhao ZM, Duan WD, Lu F, Dong JH. Robotic-assisted laparoscopic anatomic hepatectomy in China: initial experience. Ann Surg. 2011;253(2):342–8.
10. Casciola L, Patriti A, Ceccarelli G, Bartoli A, Ceribelli C, Spaziani A. Robot-assisted parenchymal-sparing liver surgery including lesions located in the posterosuperior segments. Surg Endosc. 2011;25(12):3815–24.

11. Yu HY, Friedlander DF, Patel S, Hu JC. The current status of robotic oncologic surgery. CA Cancer J Clin. 2013;63(1):45–56.
12. Buell JF, Cherqui D, Geller DA, O'Rourke N, Iannitti D, Dagher I, et al. The international position on laparoscopic liver surgery: the Louisville Statement, 2008. Ann Surg. 2009;250(5):825–30.
13. Wakabayashi G, Cherqui D, Geller DA, Buell JF, Kaneko H, Han HS, et al. Recommendations for laparoscopic liver resection: a report from the second international consensus conference held in Morioka. Ann Surg. 2015;261(4):619–29.
14. Spolverato G, Ejaz A, Kim Y, Hall BL, Bilimoria K, Cohen M, et al. Patterns of care among patients undergoing hepatic resection: a query of the National Surgical Quality Improvement Program-targeted hepatectomy database. J Surg Res. 2015;196(2):221–8.
15. Szold A, Bergamaschi R, Broeders I, Dankelman J, Forgione A, Lango T, et al. European Association of Endoscopic Surgeons (EAES) consensus statement on the use of robotics in general surgery. Surg Endosc. 2015;29(2):253–88. Epub 2014/11/09. eng.
16. Wakabayashi G, Cherqui D, Geller DA, Han HS, Kaneko H, Buell JF. Laparoscopic hepatectomy is theoretically better than open hepatectomy: preparing for the 2nd International Consensus Conference on Laparoscopic Liver Resection. J Hepatobiliary Pancreat Sci. 2014;21(10):723–31. Epub 2014/08/19. eng.
17. Li N, Wu YR, Wu B, Lu MQ. Surgical and oncologic outcomes following laparoscopic versus open liver resection for hepatocellular carcinoma: A meta-analysis. Hepatol Res. 2012;42(1):51–9.
18. Parks KR, Kuo YH, Davis JM, O'Brien B, Hagopian EJ. Laparoscopic versus open liver resection: a meta-analysis of long-term outcome. HPB (Oxford). 2014;16(2):109–18. Pubmed Central PMCID: 3921005.
19. Takahara T, Wakabayashi G, Beppu T, Aihara A, Hasegawa K, Gotohda N, et al. Long-term and perioperative outcomes of laparoscopic versus open liver resection for hepatocellular carcinoma with propensity score matching: a multi-institutional Japanese study. J Hepatobiliary Pancreat Sci. 2015;22(10):721–7.
20. Qiu J, Chen S, Chengyou D. A systematic review of robotic-assisted liver resection and meta-analysis of robotic versus laparoscopic hepatectomy for hepatic neoplasms. Surg Endosc. 2016;30(3):862–75.
21. Tsung A, Geller DA, Sukato DC, Sabbaghian S, Tohme S, Steel J, et al. Robotic versus laparoscopic hepatectomy: a matched comparison. Ann Surg. 2014;259(3):549–55.
22. Spampinato MG, Coratti A, Bianco L, Caniglia F, Laurenzi A, Puleo F, et al. Perioperative outcomes of laparoscopic and robot-assisted major hepatectomies: an Italian multi-institutional comparative study. Surg Endosc. 2014;28(10):2973–9.
23. Wu YM, Hu RH, Lai HS, Lee PH. Robotic-assisted minimally invasive liver resection. Asian J Surg. 2014;37(2):53–7.
24. Vigano L, Laurent A, Tayar C, Tomatis M, Ponti A, Cherqui D. The learning curve in laparoscopic liver resection: improved feasibility and reproducibility. Ann Surg. 2009;250(5):772–82.
25. Chen PD, Wu CY, Hu RH, Chen CN, Yuan RH, Liang JT, et al. Robotic major hepatectomy: Is there a learning curve? Surgery. 2016. Epub 2016/11/26. eng.
26. Fernandes E, Elli E, Giulianotti P. The role of the dual console in robotic surgical training. Surgery. 2014;155(1):1–4.
27. Inoue Y, Arita J, Sakamoto T, Ono Y, Takahashi M, Takahashi Y, et al. Anatomical liver resections guided by 3-dimensional parenchymal staining using fusion indocyanine green fluorescence imaging. Ann Surg. 2015;262(1):105–11. Epub 2014/06/03. eng.
28. Wottawa CR, Genovese B, Nowroozi BN, Hart SD, Bisley JW, Grundfest WS, et al. Evaluating tactile feedback in robotic surgery for potential clinical application using an animal model. Surg Endosc. 2016;30(8):3198–209. Pubmed Central PMCID: PMC4851934. Epub 2015/10/31. eng.
29. Velayutham V, Fuks D, Nomi T, Kawaguchi Y, Gayet B. 3D visualization reduces operating time when compared to high-definition 2D in laparoscopic liver resection: a case-matched study. Surg Endosc. 2016;30(1):147–53. Epub 2015/03/26. eng.
30. Chen PD, Wu CY, Hu RH, Chou WH, Lai HS, Liang JT, et al. Robotic versus open hepatectomy for hepatocellular carcinoma: a matched comparison. Ann Surg Oncol. 2016;24:1021–8. Epub 2016/10/26. eng.

# Chapter 8
# Minimally Invasive Pancreatic Surgery

Raja R. Narayan and T. Peter Kingham

## Introduction

Initial attempts at minimally invasive pancreatic operation were slow to gain traction due to lack of equipment, training, and skill [63]. Though a large incision could be avoided, this does not account for much of the morbidity associated with pancreatic surgery. Concerns were also raised that a minimally invasive approach did not allow surgeons to perform an oncologic resection with respect to margins achieved or lymph nodes retrieved. Surgical technique and training, however, have improved enabling equivalent oncologic resections. With improvements in postoperative surveillance strategies and patient management, several benefits were realized, including decreased operative blood loss and reduced hospital stay. As the volume of surgical experience grew and technology improved, a minimally invasive approach became more feasible for a variety of pancreatic diseases.

## Indications

Though a majority of pancreatic surgery is done for malignancy, several benign lesions can be resected by a minimally invasive approach.

R. R. Narayan, MD, MPH
Department of Surgery, Stanford University, Stanford, CA, USA

Department of Hepatopancreatobiliary Surgery, Memorial Sloan Kettering Cancer Center, New York City, NY, USA
e-mail: narayanr@mskcc.org

T. P. Kingham, MD (✉)
Department of Hepatopancreatobiliary Surgery, Memorial Sloan Kettering Cancer Center, New York City, NY, USA
e-mail: kinghamt@mskcc.org

© Springer Nature Switzerland AG 2019
C. Rezac, K. Donohue (eds.), *The Internist's Guide to Minimally Invasive Gastrointestinal Surgery*, Clinical Gastroenterology,
https://doi.org/10.1007/978-3-319-96631-1_8

## *Benign*

### Acute Pancreatitis

While the majority of patients that develop acute pancreatitis never require an operation, sequelae such as necrosis or pseudocyst formation can result in morbidity that warrant intervention. Operative intervention often comes at the risk of converting a sterile fluid collection or necrosum into an infected space.

Pancreatic Necrosis

Delayed surgical debridement is indicated for symptomatic sterile walled-off necrosis (WON) or infected necrosum [50]. Previously, this was done by an open approach, but cost and clinical morbidity are minimized with a minimally invasive approach [9, 10].

A step-up approach was adopted where those with suspected or confirmed infected necrosum would undergo minimally invasive retroperitoneal necrosectomy if needed after percutaneous or endoscopic drainage [71]. In doing so, control of the infectious source is prioritized over debridement of all necrotic tissue. This approach reduced cost of care as well as the need to repeat drainage or operative intervention.

With improvements in both surgical technique and inpatient care enabling delayed operative intervention, more recent studies with national database outcomes have found inpatient mortality to be less than 10% [54]. Minimally invasive debridement can be achieved by a variety of approaches (transperitoneal, retroperitoneal, peroral transmucosal, peroral transpapillary, percutaneous), methods of visualization (laparoscopic, endoscopic, radiologic, hybrid), and interventions (drainage, lavage, fragmentation, debridement, excision). A combination of patient factors, institutional experience, and surgeon preference decides which combination of approach, visualization, and intervention is employed [12]. For example, laparoscopic transgastric necrosectomy has the advantage of often requiring only a single intervention to debride infected necrosum [78]. Operative intervention, however, risks creating an enteric fistula and predisposing to pseudoaneurysmal bleed. The retroperitoneal approach, as described in the step-up approach, has been deemed safe as well, relative to open necrosectomy [33]. Peroral procedures are limited because multiple sessions are necessary for complete debridement unless a communication is made to debride into the enteric tract [70].

Pancreatic Pseudocyst

Surgical management of pancreatic pseudocysts mirrors that of necrosum but can also include laparoscopic cyst fenestration to create a conduit for drainage.

## Chronic Pancreatitis

Patients with chronic pain from long-term inflammatory obstruction of the pancreatic duct can benefit from decompression. Surgical drainage results in complete and partial pain relief more frequently than endoscopic drainage [14]. Persistent symptoms can warrant longitudinal anterior pancreaticojejunostomy (Puestow) which has been described laparoscopically [38, 39] but is usually pursued once duct stenting has failed to reduce pain. When chronic inflammatory calcification is localized at the head of the pancreas, the Frey procedure may be performed instead. Laparoscopic experience for this procedure remains relatively new as well [18].

## Cystic Neoplasm

With improved imaging, more cases of intraductal papillary mucinous neoplasms (IPMNs) are managed today with surveillance rather than surgery given the low rate of conversion to malignancy [59, 66, 72]. Figure 8.1 shows the different positions IPMNs can arise [15].

Resection is recommended for all IPMNs with solid features with a dilated pancreatic duct and/or concerning features on EUS-FNA. The recommended resection is based on the location of the IPMN along the pancreas as is done with malignant lesions (described below).

## *Malignant*

Perioperative mortality after resection of pancreatic adenocarcinoma has decreased significantly over time from improvements in critical care and inpatient management [77]. Similar to IPMNs, resection for pancreatic adenocarcinoma largely depends on the location of the tumor along the gland. A mass at the head, neck, or ampulla warrants pancreaticoduodenectomy or Whipple procedure. A mass in the body or tail generally warrants distal pancreatectomy.

## Operations

## *Diagnostic Laparoscopy*

Prior to pancreatectomy, diagnostic laparoscopy is recommended for high-risk patients to identify metastatic lesions that may preclude complete resection [45, 55]. If peritoneal or liver metastases are seen, pancreatectomy is aborted, and neoadjuvant therapy is pursued.

**Fig. 8.1** Position of IPMNs along the pancreatic duct. **a** Represents a side-branch duct IPMN. **b** Represents a main duct IPMN, *IPMN* intraductal papillary mucinous neoplasm. (Adopted from Casillas et al. [15])

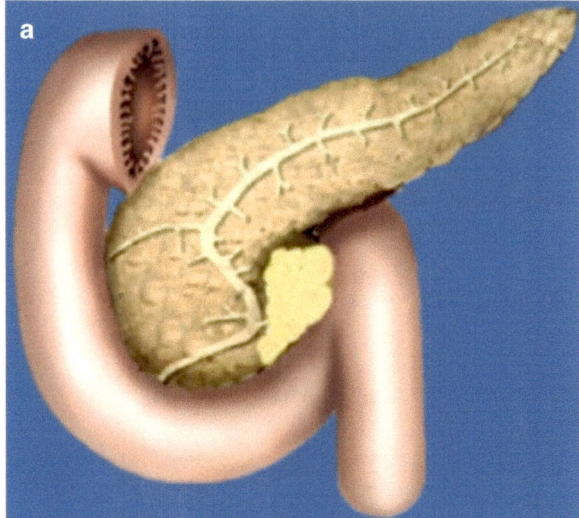

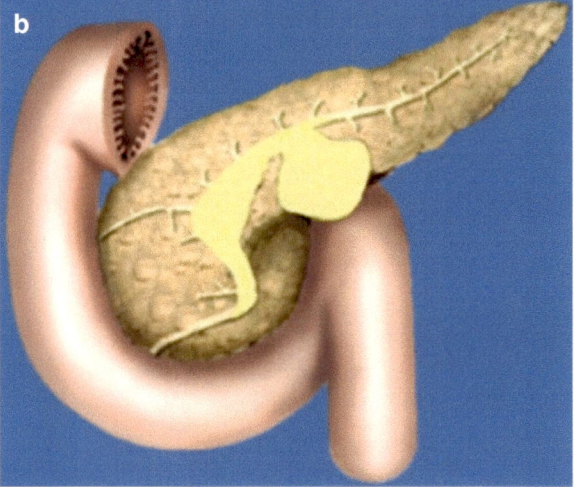

## *Distal Pancreatectomy*

In the absence of metastases, pancreatic masses along the body or tail can be resected by left or distal pancreatectomy. Since its first description in 1994 [23], use of laparoscopic distal pancreatectomy (LDP) more than tripled over the next decade [67]. In comparison with open distal pancreatectomy, LDP carries the benefit of reduced operative blood loss and need for transfusion, earlier PO tolerance, decreased length of stay, and decreased rate of wound infection [41, 46]. Studies controlling for oncologic equivalence are still pending [34, 58].

Use of three to five ports placed clockwise around the epigastrium has been described for LDP as the patient is positioned in a modified right lateral decubitus position with reverse Trendelenburg [63]. The robotic approach, first described in

2003 [32], is done similarly and has a lower incidence of conversion than LDP [25, 52]. The open approach remains the mainstay for larger tumors.

## Pancreatoduodenectomy (Whipple Procedure)

Laparoscopic pancreaticoduodenectomy (LPD) or Whipple procedure was first described in Canada [31]. Similar to LDP, LPD utilizes four to seven ports placed in a semicircle around the head of the pancreas [11]. For the operation, the patient is placed supine and in reverse Trendelenburg.

Several meta-analyses have compared LPD relative to the open approach noting decreased operative blood loss but increased operative time [21, 42, 51, 57]. More recent database studies have found higher mortality from LPD relative to the open approach at low-volume centers [60] and raise concern for increased risk of postoperative pancreatic fistula (POPF) when performed for periampullary tumors [30].

## Pancreatic Tumor Enucleation

Ectatic pancreatic masses that are distinct from the duct may be removed by enucleation. The minimally invasive approach for enucleation was described in 2011 [27]. Resistance to further adoption of this procedure is related to relatively higher rate of POPF postoperatively.

## Central Pancreatectomy

For lesions distal to the superior mesenteric vessels and away from the pancreatic tail, central pancreatectomy can be considered. Laparoscopic central pancreatectomy was first described in 2003 [5], but more widespread use of this technique has been limited by the relatively high rate of POPF [36].

## Other Operative Considerations

When the operating team presents the patient to the inpatient team for sign out, several issues should be discussed. The duration of the operation informs how long the patient underwent anesthesia and therefore sympathetic depression. Some may require intensive care unit (ICU) monitoring and vasopressors to support their circulatory system for a period of time. The volume of resuscitative fluid given intraoperatively can also contribute to whether the patient requires circulatory support postoperatively or continued ventilator support. Patients with heart failure preoperatively will be sensitive to fluid shifts and should be monitored closely as well. For several of the operations discussed, the patient should be placed in the decubitus position to aid with minimally invasive access. Though the majority of patients do well with this, some with severe joint disorders and morbid obesity can have postoperative issues that should be addressed with physical therapy and supportive care.

Finally, the surgical team will disclose if any complications or difficulties arose intraoperatively that may raise issues postoperatively. Red flags from the description of the operation include high estimated blood loss (EBL), mention of difficult dissection, and inadvertent solid or hollow viscus injury. Clear communication with the surgical team on a daily basis postoperatively is key to identifying complications immediately and managing them early.

## Postoperative Management

### Pain Control

A major advantage with minimally invasive pancreatectomy is decreased postoperative pain and narcotic requirements [3, 48]. Alhough there is no universally accepted approach to pain management for patients following minimally invasive pancreatectomy, a recent trial studying those undergoing open hepatopancreatobiliary operations supports the use of thoracic epidural analgesia over intravenous patient-controlled analgesia [2].

### Pancreatic Insufficiency

After pancreatic resection, exocrine and endocrine dyscrasias can result and must be managed to allow for optimal postoperative healing. Lack of enzyme secretion from the remnant pancreas can result in nausea, abdominal distension, and most commonly diarrhea. Exogenous pancreatic enzyme administration is needed with meals to support digestion following extensive pancreatic resection. Similarly, postpancreatectomy patients can be rendered diabetic from complete loss of insulin secretion. Early postoperative glucose monitoring is essential to determine if the patient will require insulin on an outpatient basis.

### Drain Management

There is currently no consensus on drain placement for minimally invasive pancreatectomy. Although this subject has been studied for the open approach, conflicting findings have been reported. Following pancreaticoduodenectomy, reports have shown that drain placement can predispose patients to have pancreatic fistula [1], while others report increased postoperative complications and mortality [68]. For distal pancreatectomy, no significant difference has been identified even with randomized controlled trials [69]. The ultimate decision to place a drain comes down to surgeon preference.

If a drain is placed, close daily inspection is advised to monitor for evidence of a bleed, bile leak, or pancreatic leak. Drains should be flushed two to three times daily with 10 mL of water or normal saline to prevent clogging. Most drains are removed by a member of the operative team once they collect less than 20 mL on a daily basis and the patient is doing clinically well (e.g., no fever, tachycardia, or worsening abdominal pain).

Minimal output from drains placed for known intraperitoneal collections can indicate that the fluid has been completely evacuated or that the drain is malfunctioning. If the drain is clogged, injection of tissue plasminogen activator (tPA) can break up loculations but risks an intraperitoneal bleed. Leakage of pus or fluid from around the drain can indicate it is clogged as well. If tPA is unable to unclog the drain, it can be replaced along a guidewire usually by an interventional radiologist. Conversely, ongoing high-volume output (greater than 200 mL per day) can suggest biliary, pancreatic, or enteric leak and should be further investigated (see below).

## Postoperative Complications

Whether minimally invasive or open, pancreatectomy carries significant risks for many postoperative complications such as pneumonia, urinary tract infection, septicemia, venous thromboembolism, pulmonary embolism, arrhythmia, and myocardial infarction [49]. A hospitalist managing pancreatectomy patients postoperatively must be well-versed in the management of these issues as well as those complications specific to the procedure, as summarized in Table 8.1.

### *Hemorrhage*

The presentation for postoperative hemorrhage can be heterogeneous due to multiple possible sources for a bleed. To determine next steps of management, it is best to classify postoperative hemorrhage using a standard definition (Table 8.2).

The source of postoperative bleeding is a critical determinant for management strategy. Location is broadly divided into intraluminal and extraluminal. Intraluminal sources of hemorrhage can include the anastomotic site, the interface of the pancreas to the anastomosing biliary or enteric tract, stress ulcers, and pseudoaneurysms. Extraluminal bleeds can originate from the resection bed, suture line, and pseudoaneurysms as well.

The timing of a postoperative bleed also determines the invasiveness of the indicated management. Early bleeding (within 24 hours of initial pancreatectomy) is

**Table 8.1** Common complications associated with minimally invasive pancreatectomy

| Study | N | SSI | Intra-abdominal collection | Fistula | Hemorrhage | DGE | Reoperation | Death |
|---|---|---|---|---|---|---|---|---|
| *Laparoscopic pancreaticoduodenectomy* | | | | | | | | |
| Palanivelu et al. [53] | 42 | – | 2 (5%) | 3 (7%) | – | 1 (2%) | 1 (2%) | 1 (2%) |
| Kendrick et al. [37] | 62 | 4 (6%) | – | 11 (18%) | 5 (8%) | 9 (15%) | 3 (5%) | 1 (2%) |
| Zureikat et al. [83] | 14 | 3 (21%) | – | 5 (36%) | 2 (14%) | 3 (21%) | 1 (7%) | 1 (7%) |
| Asbun et al. [4] | 53 | 6 (11%) | 10 (19%) | 7 (13%) | 5 (9%) | 6 (11%) | 2 (4%) | 3 (6%) |
| Corcione et al. [19] | 22 | – | 2 (9%) | 6 (27%) | 5 (23%) | – | 3 (14%) | 1 (5%) |
| Croome et al. [22] | 108 | – | – | 12 (11%) | 8 (7%) | 10 (9%) | – | 1 (1%) |
| Dokmak et al. [30] | 46 | – | 5 (11%) | 22 (48%) | 11 (24%) | 8 (17%) | 11 (24%) | 1 (2%) |
| Tan et al. [65] | 30 | – | 1 (3%) | 10 (33%) | 1 (3%) | 2 (7%) | – | – |
| Delitto et al. [28] | 52 | 8 (15%) | – | 9 (17%) | 5 (10%) | – | – | 1 (2%) |
| Chapman et al. [16] | 22 | 2 (9%) | 2 (9%) | 8 (36%) | – | 6 (27%) | – | 0 (0%) |
| Stauffer et al. [64] | 58 | 5 (9%) | – | 6 (10%) | 4 (7%) | 10 (17%) | 1 (2%) | 2 (3%) |
| *Laparoscopic distal pancreatectomy* | | | | | | | | |
| DiNorcia et al. [29] | 71 | – | – | 8 (11%) | – | – | 4 (6%) | 0 (0%) |
| Butturini et al. [13] | 43 | – | 8 (19%) | 12 (28%) | 4 (9%) | – | 4 (9%) | 0 (0%) |
| Cho et al. [17] | 254 | 9 (4%) | 1 (6%) | 57 (22%) | – | – | 3 (1%) | 1 (<0.01%) |
| Limongelli et al. [43] | 16 | 2 (13%) | 1 (6%) | 3 (19%) | 0 (0%) | 1 (6%) | 0 (0%) | 0 (0%) |
| Mehta et al. [47] | 30 | – | 6 (20%) | 5 (17%) | – | – | 1 (3%) | 0 (0%) |
| Baker et al. [6] | 48 | 6 (13%) | – | 27 (56%) | – | 4 (8%) | – | 2 (4%) |
| Zhang et al. [81] | 20 | – | 0 (0%) | 5 (25%) | – | 0 (0%) | – | 0 (0%) |
| Lee et al. [41] | 131 | – | 14 (11%) | 11 (8%) | – | – | – | 0 (0%) |
| de Rooij et al. [26] | 63 | 5 (8%) | 4 (6%) | 7 (11%) | 1 (2%) | 3 (5%) | – | 2 (3%) |
| Joliat et al. [35] | 26 | – | – | 5 (19%) | 2 (8%) | – | – | 0 (0%) |
| Stauffer et al. [62] | 44 | 4 (9%) | 3 (7%) | 6 (14%) | 1 (2%) | – | 1 (2%) | 1 (2%) |
| Xourafas et al. [79] | 694 | 19 (3%) | 49 (7%) | 128 (18%) | 37 (5%) | 22 (3%) | 23 (3%) | 8 (1%) |
| *Laparoscopic central pancreatectomy* | | | | | | | | |
| Song et al. [61] | 26 | – | – | 5 (19%) | – | – | 0 (0%) | 0 (0%) |
| Zhang et al. [82] | 17 | – | 3 (18%) | 10 (59%) | 4 (24%) | 1 (6%) | 4 (24%) | 0 (0%) |

**Table 8.2** International Study Group of Pancreatic Surgery (ISGPS) classification of postpancreatectomy hemorrhage

| Clinical variables | Grade A | Grade B | Grade C |
|---|---|---|---|
| Onset | Early | Early or late | Early or late |
| Location | Intra- or extraluminal | Intra- or extraluminal | Intra- or extraluminal |
| Clinical condition | Well | Well, intermediate | Poor, impaired |
| Management | Observation | Transfusion Endoscopy Embolization Reoperation if early | Transfer to ICU Transfusion Angiography Endoscopy Embolization Reoperation |

Adopted from Wente et al. [75]
*ICU* intensive care unit

more likely from technical failure to achieve hemostasis intraoperatively and may better benefit from reoperation [74]. Late bleeding (24 hours or more after initial pancreatectomy) may occur from postoperative inflammation leading to an anastomotic ulcer, abscess, leak, or fistula [20]. Early bleeding is often from an extraluminal source, while late bleeding tends to have intraluminal etiology. A patient with late bleeding should generally be immediately evaluated with an angiogram by interventional radiology.

The severity of postoperative bleeding can be described based on hemoglobin drop (mild if $\leq 3$ g/dL or severe if $>3$ g/dL) or the amount of products transfused (mild if $\leq 3$u packed red blood cells or severe if $>3$u packed red blood cells). A grading scheme is also available to guide therapy with severity of bleeding ranging from A (mild) to C (severe).

Imaging can aid in the localization of hemorrhage. Computed tomography (CT) with angiography is ideal for identifying if there is active extravasation from an arterial source. This can aid in delineating whether management needs to be supportive, operative, or by percutaneous embolization. A pseudoaneurysm can also be the culprit of a bleed and is identified as an enhancing structure on CT that maintains its shape in delayed phases. More often, pseudoaneurysms are best managed with embolization or placement of a covered metal stent.

## Intra-abdominal Fluid Collection

A variety of collections can develop within the abdomen postoperatively. After every pancreatic resection, there is some fluid present, most often simple fluid. Imaging can be useful to inform the next step in management if a patient has symptoms and a fluid collection. Rim enhancement around a fluid collection can suggest the presence of an abscess warranting antibiotics and possible drain placement. Gas formation within fluid can be seen in the context of infection or enteric leak. If an enteric leak is suspected, administration of oral contrast prior to imaging is useful for identifying a location for extravasation. A pancreatic or biliary leak is more challenging to identify solely on the basis of imaging.

Further delineating the source of a collection can be done with laboratory analysis of drain fluid including Gram stain with culture (for abscess or enteric leak), measurement of amylase (pancreatic leak), or total bilirubin (bile leak).

## Pancreatic Leak and Fistula

If there is concern for pancreatic leak, drain placement, while indicated, would yield serous or serosanguinous fluid resembling peritoneal fluid. Instead, fluid amylase should be compared to serum levels. A pancreatic leak is defined as the presence of a fluid collection for which fluid amylase content is at least threefold greater than serum amylase on or after postoperative day 3 [7]. A pancreatic leak can occur from breakdown of a pancreatogastrostomy or pancreatojejunostomy, but fluid may also leak from a distal pancreatectomy stump. Over time, a POPF can form if a drain is in place or if a communication between the leak and the skin forms. POPF is the most common serious complication following pancreatectomy. Suspicion for POPF should be raised with any abdominal discomfort, nausea, tachycardia, or fever. Once identified, POPF is graded based on its severity, as shown in Table 8.3.

This grading system has been validated showing that patients who develop a Grade A POPF tend to have shorter length of stay (LOS) and fewer secondary complications than more severe fistulae [56].

**Table 8.3** International Study Group of Pancreatic Fistula (ISGPF) grading

| Clinical variables | Grade A | Grade B | Grade C |
|---|---|---|---|
| Condition | Well | Usually well | Appears ill |
| Requires supportive therapy[a] | − | ± | + |
| Imaging findings | − | ± | + |
| Drainage persists ≥3 weeks[b] | − | ± | + |
| Signs of infection | − | + | + |
| Sepsis | − | − | + |
| Readmission | − | ± | ± |
| Reoperation | − | − | + |
| Death resulting from fistula | − | − | + |

Adopted from Bassi et al. [7]
[a]Can include critical care admission, receipt of antibiotics, somatostatin analogue, peripheral parenteral nutrition (PPN), total parenteral nutrition (TPN), or enteric nutrition
[b]Drain does not need to be in place to qualify

Management of POPF involves adequate drainage and limiting stimulation of the pancreas beginning with restriction of oral intake. If drainage persists despite this, the patient may require nutritional support by TPN or enteral feeding distal to the duodenum. As mentioned earlier, support with enteral feeding is superior to TPN resulting in more frequent and rapid closure of POPF [40]. TPN additionally carries the risk of line sepsis, metabolite derangement, cirrhosis, and enteric atrophy. There is also data supporting the use of long-lasting somatostatin analogues (e.g., pasire-otide) to prevent the incidence of POPF when started preoperatively; however, more data is needed to support its use if initiated postoperatively [1]. Most fistulae, up to 90%, will spontaneously close in 4 weeks [44]. Ultimate resolution of POPF is done on an outpatient basis.

## Biliary Leak, Stricture, or Infection

A biliary leak may be discovered earlier than pancreatic leak due to the distinct green color of the fluid. If still equivocal, fluid total bilirubin can be compared to serum levels. A fivefold increase in fluid bilirubin compared to serum is indicative of bile leak [24]. Intraperitoneal leakage of bile can result in fluid collections that may become infected or cause bile peritonitis. If not already present, drain place-ment is indicated to control the leak. Small leaks have the potential to resolve spon-taneously [73]. Complete bile duct transection, however, requires operative intervention. Persistent drainage of more than 100 mL of bile daily can result in metabolite derangements and dehydration. At this point, percutaneous or endo-scopic diversion of bile away from the defect is needed to decompress the biliary tree and heal the site of leakage. This can be achieved by percutaneous transhepatic biliary drainage (PTBD) or endoscopic stenting across or excluding the defect.

Biliary stricture, in the context of pancreatic surgery, occurs at the bilioenteric anastomosis (hepaticojejunostomy or choledochojejunostomy). This may initially manifest with abdominal distension or discomfort, nausea, or jaundice. Following biliary dissection and instrumentation, a high level of suspicion should also exist for cholangitis which may present with similar symptoms including fever, right upper quadrant pain, jaundice, altered mental status, and eventually hypotension. The workup of biliary strictures should rule out cholangitis.

Balloon cholangioplasty or stent placement across a stricture should be attempted to reconstitute flow. If unsuccessful, an internal-external biliary drain can be placed to decompress the biliary tree. These drains have holes that are positioned on either side of the obstruction to allow bile to circumvent the stricture and drain into either the enteric tract or an external bag. The drain can be "capped" if the patient is clini-cally doing well and the output is not significantly bloody to allow bile to drain solely into the enteric tract. Most patients with bile leaks or biliary strictures are discharged with at least one drain in place for continued decompression until the drain can be removed on an outpatient basis.

**Table 8.4** ISGPS grading of delayed gastric emptying severity

| Clinical variables | Grade A | Grade B | Grade C |
|---|---|---|---|
| Vomiting or distension | ± | + | + |
| Duration NPO | POD 7 | POD 14 | POD 21 |
| NGT use | ≤POD 7 or reinsertion > POD 3 | POD 8–14 or reinsertion > POD 7 | >POD 14 or reinsertion > POD 14 |
| Prokinetic use | ± | + | + |

Adopted from Wente et al. [76]
*ISGPS* International Study Group of Pancreatic Surgery, *NPO* non per os, *NGT* nasogastric tube, *POD* postoperative day

## Delayed Gastric Emptying

Following upper gastrointestinal surgery, functional gastroparesis can result in the absence of mechanical obstruction. This can manifest as nausea, vomiting, and abdominal distension. Delayed gastric emptying (DGE) should be confirmed by ruling out a mechanical small bowel obstruction or anastomotic stricture using an upper GI contrast series or endoscopy [76]. While the etiology of DGE remains elusive, it is believed that decreased motilin release from enterochromaffin cells contributes to its occurrence [80]. Additionally, secondary causes such as POPF or intraperitoneal fluid collections can predispose to its occurrence [8]. Similar to other postpancreatectomy complications, DGE has a formal severity classification system to report and analyze its incidence across institutions (Table 8.4).

Management of DGE begins with restricting diet to prevent worsening nausea or distension. If nausea or vomiting persists, a nasogastric tube (NGT) can be placed to decompress the upper GI tract. Following decompression, if motility is not regained, then a prokinetic agent can be administered. Erythromycin is a prokinetic agent which acts as a motilin receptor agonist and has been shown to decrease the incidence of DGE, need for NGT reinsertion, and time to tolerating PO [80]. If patients fail to improve with NPO, NGT, and prokinetic agents, nutritional support is needed. For those unable to attain regular diet by 7–10 days, starting nutritional support has been shown to result in regular diet tolerance earlier and reduced readmission rate [8]. As noted earlier, enteric nutrition should be prioritized over parenteral. Finally, imaging may be required to look for secondary causes of DGE. Presence of an intraperitoneal collection or POPF can necessitate drain placement as other more supportive strategies may fail to resolve DGE.

## Conclusion

Similar to open procedures, minimally invasive pancreatectomy carries the risk of significant postoperative morbidity. This requires close patient monitoring.

Ultimately, communication and strategizing between the surgical internist and operative team are essential for early detection and mitigation of complications before clinical deterioration can take hold.

# References

1. Allen PJ. Pasireotide for postoperative pancreatic fistula. N Engl J Med. 2014;371:875–6.
2. Aloia TA, Kim BJ, Segraves-Chun YS, et al. A randomized controlled trial of postoperative thoracic epidural analgesia versus intravenous patient-controlled analgesia after major hepatopancreatobiliary surgery. Ann Surg. 2017;266(3):545–54.
3. Aly MY, Tsutsumi K, Nakamura M, et al. Comparative study of laparoscopic and open distal pancreatectomy. J Laparoendosc Adv Surg Tech A. 2010;20:435–40.
4. Asbun HJ, Stauffer JA. Laparoscopic vs open pancreaticoduodenectomy: overall outcomes and severity of complications using the Accordion Severity Grading System. J Am Coll Surg. 2012;215(6):810–9.
5. Baca I, Bokan I. Laparoscopic segmental pancreas resection and pancreatic cystadenoma. Chirurg. 2003;74(10):961–5.
6. Baker MS, Sherman KL, Stocker S, et al. Defining quality for distal pancreatectomy: does the laparoscopic approach protect patients from poor quality outcomes? J Gastrointest Surg. 2013;17(2):273–80.
7. Bassi C, et al. Postoperative pancreatic fistula: an international study group (ISGPF) definition. Surgery. 2005;138(1):8–13.
8. Beane JD, et al. Optimal management of delayed gastric emptying after pancreatectomy: an analysis of 1,089 patients. Surgery. 2014;156(4):939–46.
9. Besselink MG, de Bruijn MT, Rutten JP, et al. Surgical intervention in patients with necrotizing pancreatitis. Br J Surg. 2006a;93(5):593–9.
10. Besselink MG, van Santvoort HC, Nieuwenhuijs VB, et al. Minimally invasive 'step-up approach' versus maximal necrosectomy in patients with acute necrotising pancreatitis (PANTER trial): design and rationale of a randomised controlled multicenter trial. BMC Surg. 2006b;6:6.
11. Boggi U, Amorese G, Vistoli F, et al. Laparoscopic pancreaticoduodenectomy: a systematic literature review. Surg Endosc. 2015;29(1):9–23.
12. Bugiantella W, Rondelli F, Boni M, et al. Necrotizing pancreatitis: a review of the interventions. Int J Surg. 2016;28(Suppl 1):S163–71.
13. Butturini G, Partelli S, Crippa S, et al. Perioperative and long-term results after left pancreatectomy: a single-institution, non-randomized, comparative study between open and laparoscopic approach. Surg Endosc. 2011;25(9):2871–8.
14. Cahen DL, Gouma DJ, Nio Y, et al. Endoscopic versus surgical drainage of the pancreatic duct in chronic pancreatitis. N Engl J Med. 2007;356(7):676–84.
15. Casillas J, Levi JU, Garcia-Buitrago MT, Quiroz A, Ribeiro A. Intraductal papillary mucinous neoplasm (IPMN). In: Casillas J, Levi JU, Quiroz A, Ruiz-Cordero R, Garcia-Buitrago MT, Sleeman D, editors. Multidisciplinary teaching atlas of the pancreas. 1st ed. Springer: New York; 2016.
16. Chapman BC, Gleisner A, Ibrahim-Zada I, et al. Laparoscopic pancreaticoduodenectomy: changing the management of ampullary neoplasms. Surg Endosc. 2017;32:915–22. https://doi.org/10.1007/s00464-017-5766-8.
17. Cho CS, Kooby DA, Schmidt CM, et al. Laparoscopic versus open left pancreatectomy: can preoperative factors indicate the safer technique? Ann Surg. 2011;253(5):975–80.
18. Cooper MA, Datta TS, Makary MA. Laparoscopic frey procedure for chronic pancreatitis. Surg Laparosc Endosc Percutan Tech. 2014;24(1):e16–20.

19. Corcione F, Pirozzi F, Cuccurullo D, et al. Laparoscopic pancreaticoduodenectomy: experience of 22 cases. Surg Endosc. 2013;27(6):2131–6.
20. Correa-Gallego C, Brennan MF, D'Angelica MI, et al. Contemporary experience with postpancreatectomy hemorrhage: results of 1,122 patients resected between 2006 and 2011. J Am Coll Surg. 2012;215(5):616–21.
21. Correa-Gallego C, Dinkelspiel HE, Sulimanoff I, et al. Minimally-invasive vs open pancreaticoduodenectomy: systematic review and meta-analysis. J Am Coll Surg. 2014;218(1):129–39.
22. Croome KP, Farnell MB, Que FG, et al. Total laparoscopic pancreaticoduodenectomy for pancreatic ductal adenocarcinoma: oncologic advantages over open approaches? Ann Surg. 2014;260(4):633–8; discussion 638–40.
23. Cuschieri A. Laparoscopic surgery of the pancreas. J R Coll Surg Edinb. 1994;39:178–84.
24. Darwin P, et al. Jackson Pratt drain fluid-to-serum bilirubin concentration ratio for the diagnosis of bile leaks. Gastrointest Endosc. 2010;71(1):99–104.
25. Daouadi M, Zureikat AH, Zenati MS, et al. Robot-assisted minimally invasive distal pancreatectomy is superior to the laparoscopic technique. Ann Surg. 2013;257(1):128–32.
26. de Rooij T, Jilesen AP, Boerma D, et al. A nationwide comparison of laparoscopic and open distal pancreatectomy for benign and malignant disease. J Am Coll Surg. 2015;220(3):263–270.e1.
27. Dedieu A, Rault A, Collet D, et al. Laparoscopic enucleation of pancreatic neoplasm. Surg Endosc. 2011;25(2):572–6.
28. Delitto D, Luckhurst CM, Black BS, et al. Oncologic and perioperative outcomes following selective application of laparoscopic pancreaticoduodenectomy for periampullary malignancies. J Gastrointest Surg. 2016;20(7):1343–9.
29. DiNorcia J, Schrope BA, Lee MK, et al. Laparoscopic distal pancreatectomy offers shorter hospital stays with fewer complications. J Gastrointest Surg. 2010;14(11):1804–12.
30. Dokmak S, Ftériche FS, Aussilhou B, et al. Laparoscopic pancreaticoduodenectomy should not be routine for resection of periampullary tumors. J Am Coll Surg. 2015;220(5):831–8.
31. Gagner M, Pomp A. Laparoscopic pylorus-preserving pancreatoduodenectomy. Surg Endosc. 1994;8(5):408–10.
32. Giulianotti PC, Coratti A, Angelini M, et al. Robotics in general surgery: personal experience in a large community hospital. Arch Surg. 2003;138:777–84.
33. Horvath K, Freeny P, Escallon J, et al. Safety and efficacy of video-assisted retroperitoneal debridement for infected pancreatic collections: a multicenter, prospective, single-arm phase 2 study. Arch Surg. 2010;145:817–25.
34. Huang B, Feng L, Zhao J. Systematic review and meta-analysis of robotic versus laparoscopic distal pancreatectomy for benign and malignant pancreatic lesions. Surg Endosc. 2016;30(9):4078–85.
35. Joliat GR, Demartines N, Halkic N, et al. Short-term outcomes after distal pancreatectomy: laparotomy vs. laparoscopy – a single-center series. Ann Med Surg (Lond). 2016;13:1–5.
36. Kang CM, Lee JH, Lee WJ. Minimally invasive central pancreatectomy: current status and future directions. J Hepatobiliary Pancreat Sci. 2014;21(12):831–40.
37. Kendrick ML, Cusati D. Total laparoscopic pancreaticoduodenectomy: feasibility and outcome in an early experience. Arch Surg. 2010;145(1):19–23.
38. Khaled YS, Ammori BJ. Laparoscopic lateral pancreaticojejunostomy and laparoscopic Berne modification of Beger procedure for the treatment of chronic pancreatitis: the first UK experience. Surg Laparosc Endosc Percutan Tech. 2014;24(5):e178–82.
39. Kim EY, Hong TH. Laparoscopic longitudinal pancreaticojejunostomy using barbed sutures: an efficient and secure solution for pancreatic duct obstructions in patients with chronic pancreatitis. J Gastrointest Surg. 2016;20(4):861–6.
40. Klek S, et al. Enteral and parenteral nutrition in the conservative treatment of pancreatic fistula: a randomized clinical trial. Gastroenterology. 2011;141(1):157–63, 163.e1.
41. Lee SY, Allen PJ, Sadot E, et al. Distal pancreatectomy: a single institution's experience in open, laparoscopic, and robotic approaches. J Am Coll Surg. 2015;220(1):18–27.

42. Lei P, Wei B, Guo W, et al. Minimally invasive surgical approach compared with open pancreaticoduodenectomy: a systematic review and meta-analysis on the feasibility and safety. Surg Laparosc Endosc Percutan Tech. 2014;24(4):296–305.
43. Limongelli P, Belli A, Russo G, et al. Laparoscopic and open surgical treatment of left-sided pancreatic lesions: clinical outcomes and cost-effectiveness analysis. Surg Endosc. 2012;26(7):1830–6.
44. Machado NO. Pancreatic fistula after pancreatectomy: definitions, risk factors, preventive measures, and management—review. Int J Surg. 2012:602478.
45. Maithel SK, Maloney S, Winston C, et al. Preoperative CA 19-9 and the yield of staging laparoscopy in patients with radiographically resectable pancreatic adenocarcinoma. Ann Surg Oncol. 2008;15(12):3512–20.
46. Mehrabi A, Hafezi M, Arvin J, et al. A systematic review and meta-analysis of laparoscopic versus open distal pancreatectomy for benign and malignant lesions of the pancreas: it's time to randomize. Surgery. 2015;157(1):45–55.
47. Mehta SS, Doumane G, Mura T, et al. Laparoscopic versus open distal pancreatectomy: a single-institution case-control study. Surg Endosc. 2012;26(2):402–7.
48. Merkow J, Paniccia A, Edil BH. Laparoscopic pancreaticoduodenectomy: a descriptive and comparative review. Chin J Cancer Res. 2015;27:368–75.
49. Mezhir JJ. Management of complications following pancreatic resection: an evidence-based approach. J Surg Oncol. 2013;107(1):58–66.
50. Mier J, León EL, Castillo A, et al. Early versus late necrosectomy in severe necrotizing pancreatitis. Am J Surg. 1997;173:71–5.
51. Nigri GR, Rosman AS, Petrucciani N, et al. Metaanalysis of trials comparing minimally invasive and open distal pancreatectomies. Surg Endosc. 2011;25(5):1642–51.
52. Ntourakis D, Marzano E, Lopez Penza PA, et al. Robotic distal splenopancreatectomy: bridging the gap between pancreatic and minimal access surgery. J Gastrointest Surg. 2010;14(8):1326–30.
53. Palanivelu C, Jani K, Senthilnathan P, et al. Laparoscopic pancreaticoduodenectomy: technique and outcomes. J Am Coll Surg. 2007;205(2):222–30.
54. Parikh PY, Pitt HA, Kilbane M, et al. Pancreatic necrosectomy: North American mortality is much lower than expected. J Am Coll Surg. 2009;209(6):712–9.
55. Pisters PW, Lee JE, Vauthey JN, et al. Laparoscopy in the staging of pancreatic cancer. Br J Surg. 2001;88(3):325–37.
56. Pratt W, et al. Postoperative pancreatic fistulas are not equivalent after proximal, distal, and central pancreatectomy. J Gastrointest Surg. 2006;10(9):1264–78, discussion 1278–1279.
57. Qin H, Qiu J, Zhao Y, et al. Does minimally-invasive pancreaticoduodenectomy have advantages over its open method? A meta-analysis of retrospective studies. PLoS One. 2014;9(8):e104274.
58. Riviere D, Gurusamy KS, Kooby DA, et al. Laparoscopic versus open distal pancreatectomy for pancreatic cancer. Cochrane Database Syst Rev. 2016;4:CD011391.
59. Rodriguez JR, Salvia R, Crippa S, et al. Branch-duct intraductal papillary mucinous neoplasms: observations in 145 patients who underwent resection. Gastroenterology. 2007;133:72–9.
60. Sharpe SM, Talamonti MS, Wang CE, et al. Early national experience with laparoscopic pancreaticoduodenectomy for ductal adenocarcinoma: a comparison of laparoscopic pancreaticoduodenectomy and open pancreaticoduodenectomy from the national cancer data base. Am Coll Surg. 2015;221(1):175–84.
61. Song KB, Kim SC, Park KM, et al. Laparoscopic central pancreatectomy for benign or low-grade malignant lesions in the pancreatic neck and proximal body. Surg Endosc. 2015;29(4):937–46.
62. Stauffer JA, Coppola A, Mody K, et al. Laparoscopic versus open distal pancreatectomy for pancreatic adenocarcinoma. World J Surg. 2016;40(6):1477–84.
63. Stauffer JA, Asbun HJ. Minimally invasive pancreatic resectional techniques. In: Jarnagin WR, editor. Blumgart's surgery of the liver, pancreas, and biliary tract. 6th ed. Philadelphia: Elsevier; 2017.

64. Stauffer JA, Coppola A, Villacreses D, et al. Laparoscopic versus open pancreaticoduodenectomy for pancreatic adenocarcinoma: long-term results at a single institution. Surg Endosc. 2017;31(5):2233–41.
65. Tan CL, Zhang H, Peng B, et al. Outcome and costs of laparoscopic pancreaticoduodenectomy during the initial learning curve vs laparotomy. World J Gastroenterol. 2015;21(17):5311–9.
66. Tanaka M, Cahri S, Adsay V, et al. International consensus guidelines for management of intraductal papillary mucinous neoplasms and mucinous cystic neoplasms of the pancreas. Pancreatology. 2006;6:17–32.
67. Tran Cao HS, Lopez N, Chang DC, et al. Improved perioperative outcomes with minimally invasive distal pancreatectomy: results from a population-based analysis. JAMA Surg. 2014;149(3):237–43.
68. Van Buren G 2nd, Bloomston M, Hughes SJ, et al. A randomized prospective multicenter trial of pancreaticoduodenectomy with and without routine intraperitoneal drainage. Ann Surg. 2014;259(4):605–12.
69. Van Buren G 2nd, Bloomston M, Schmidt CR, et al. A prospective randomized multicenter trial of distal pancreatectomy with and without routine intraperitoneal drainage. Ann Surg. 2017;266(3):421–31.
70. van Grinsven J, van Santvoort HC, Boermeester MA, et al. Timing of catheter drainage in infected necrotizing pancreatitis. Nat Rev Gastroenterol Hepatol. 2016;13(5):306–12.
71. van Santvoort HC, Besselink MG, Bakker OJ, et al. A step-up approach or open necrosectomy for necrotizing pancreatitis. N Engl J Med. 2010;362(16):1491–502.
72. Vege SS, Ziring B, Jain R, Moayyedi P, Clinical Guidelines Committee, American Gastroenterology Association. American gastroenterological association institute guideline on the diagnosis and management of asymptomatic neoplastic pancreatic cysts. Gastroenterology. 2015;148(4):819.
73. Viganò L, et al. Bile leak after hepatectomy: predictive factors of spontaneous healing. Am J Surg. 2008;196(2):195–200.
74. Wellner UF, et al. Postpancreatectomy hemorrhage–incidence, treatment, and risk factors in over 1,000 pancreatic resections. J Gastrointest Surg. 2014;18(3):464–75.
75. Wente MN, et al. Postpancreatectomy hemorrhage (PPH): an international study group of pancreatic surgery (ISGPS) definition. Surgery. 2007a;142(1):20–5.
76. Wente MN, et al. Delayed gastric emptying (DGE) after pancreatic surgery: a suggested definition by the International Study Group of Pancreatic Surgery (ISGPS). Surgery. 2007b;142(5):761–8.
77. Winter JM, Brennan MF, Tang LH, et al. Survival after resection of pancreatic adenocarcinoma: results from a single institution over three decades. Ann Surg Oncol. 2012;19(1):169–75.
78. Worhunsky DJ, Qadan M, Dua MM, et al. Laparoscopic transgastric necrosectomy for the management of pancreatic necrosis. J Am Coll Surg. 2014;219(4):735–43.
79. Xourafas D, Ashley SW, Clancy TE. Comparison of perioperative outcomes between open, laparoscopic, and robotic distal pancreatectomy: an analysis of 1815 patients from the ACS-NSQIP procedure-targeted pancreatectomy database. J Gastrointest Surg. 2017;21:1442–52. https://doi.org/10.1007/s11605-017-3463-5.
80. Yeo CJ, et al. Erythromycin accelerates gastric emptying after pancreaticoduodenectomy. A prospective, randomized, placebo-controlled trial. Ann Surg. 1993;218(3):229–37, discussion 237–238.
81. Zhang Y, Chen XM, Sun DL. Laparoscopic versus open distal pancreatectomy: a single-institution comparative study. World J Surg Oncol. 2014;12:327.
82. Zhang RC, Zhang B, Mou YP, et al. Comparison of clinical outcomes and quality of life between laparoscopic and open central pancreatectomy with pancreaticojejunostomy. Surg Endosc. 2017;31:4756. https://doi.org/10.1007/s00464-017-5552-7.
83. Zureikat AH, Breaux JA, Steel JL, et al. Can laparoscopic pancreaticoduodenectomy be safely implemented? J Gastrointest Surg. 2011;15(7):1151–7.

# Chapter 9
# Minimally Invasive Small Bowel Surgery

**Jessica S. Crystal and Miral Sadaria Grandhi**

## Introduction

Minimally invasive surgery has been growing in favor over the past several decades, and it has been proven to be safe and feasible for organs beyond just the gallbladder, particularly the small intestine [1]. While the laparoscopic approach has been accepted as the standard of care for cholecystectomy, a consensus has not been reached for surgery of the small intestinal tract [2]. Some of the benefits demonstrated for laparoscopic surgery compared to open surgery include reduced postoperative complications (including wound infections), decreased incidence of hernias, improved cosmetic results, improved postoperative recovery, decreased intraoperative and postoperative pain, quicker return of bowel function, shorter length of stay, faster return to normal activity and diet, improved social and sexual interaction, and decreased rate of adhesive small bowel obstruction [2–5]. These procedures are similar to those performed during open surgery but require the surgeon to translate the same principles to a confined space, often maneuvering longer instruments in technically challenging angles. The indications for these procedures are similar to the open approach, including both benign and malignant processes, and are being performed in elective, urgent, and even trauma settings [6, 7].

J. S. Crystal
Department of Surgery, Rutgers Robert Wood Johnson Medical School,
New Brunswick, NJ, USA

M. S. Grandhi (✉)
Department of Surgery, Rutgers Robert Wood Johnson Medical School,
New Brunswick, NJ, USA

Department of Surgery, Division of Surgical Oncology, Rutgers Cancer Institute of New Jersey, New Brunswick, NJ, USA
e-mail: miral.grandhi@rutgers.edu

© Springer Nature Switzerland AG 2019
C. Rezac, K. Donohue (eds.), *The Internist's Guide to Minimally Invasive Gastrointestinal Surgery*, Clinical Gastroenterology,
https://doi.org/10.1007/978-3-319-96631-1_9

The evolution of minimally invasive techniques for small bowel surgery started with the success of the laparoscopic approach to disease processes of the appendix and colon. The first laparoscopic appendectomy was performed by Kurt Semm in 1983 [4]. Laparoscopic techniques were then applied to colon surgery with the first laparoscopic right hemicolectomy performed by Moises Jacobs in June of 1990 in Miami, Florida. Subsequently, the first entirely laparoscopic right hemicolectomy with an intracorporeal ileocolonic anastomosis was performed on July 26, 1991, by Joseph Uddo [8]. Further contributions included the first reported successful laparoscopic adhesiolysis in 1991 by Bastug et al. [9]. Over the next three decades, the minimally invasive approach to small bowel surgery was applied more broadly with the use of laparoscopy for many other benign diseases, including Crohn's disease, Meckel's diverticulum, superior mesenteric artery (SMA) syndrome, intussusception, gallstone ileus, foreign body removal, and almost any other disease entity in which open surgery has been indicated [1, 10–12]. Likewise, laparoscopy has also been utilized safely in the management of many malignancies requiring surgical intervention, including gastrointestinal stromal tumors (GIST), neuroendocrine tumors (NET), lymphoma, lipoma, schwannoma, sarcoma, adenocarcinoma, and other tumors found in the small intestine as well as for the identification of metastatic disease with diagnostic laparoscopy [1, 13–16]. Additionally, laparoscopy can be useful for diagnosing the etiology of abdominal pain of unknown origin [17]. With the advent of robotic surgery, surgeons are increasingly performing small intestinal surgery robotically; however, the studies examining the safety of robotic small bowel surgery are limited to some case series and reports [18].

## Preoperative Considerations

When anticipating a minimally invasive approach to small bowel surgery, many of the same principles should be adhered to as in an open case. These include a full history and physical examination, including a review of systems. Appropriate laboratory testing, including CBC, BMP, hepatic function panel, coagulation panel, lactate, and/or arterial blood gas, may be useful in assessing the patient and narrowing down the differential diagnoses further. Imaging with x-ray, ultrasound, cross-sectional imaging, and/or other studies can be useful, particularly when planning for a minimally invasive approach. These studies can help assess the appropriateness of approaching the case in a minimally invasive fashion and provide a road map for the surgeon in regard to the anatomy. The details of the diagnostic work-up of each of these disease processes are beyond the scope of this chapter and can be reviewed in other texts.

## Indications and Outcomes in Laparoscopic Small Bowel Surgery

With the increased training and comfort in advanced laparoscopic techniques among surgeons, the use of laparoscopy for small intestine pathology has been growing

[19]. To follow is a more detailed review of the progression of minimally invasive techniques for a variety of small bowel disorders.

## Small Bowel Obstruction

Small bowel obstruction is a disease process that is often managed non-operatively, but when operative intervention is required, surgeons traditionally approach this process with an open surgical procedure. The default to an open operation is often due to the concern for inadequate intra-abdominal working space to visualize the pathology secondary to dilated loops of small bowel as well as the concern for possible injury to dilated and friable loops of small bowel. The laparoscopic approach to lysis of adhesions was first described for the treatment of chronic pelvic pain and infertility by gynecologists in the 1970s [20]. This technique was first applied to small bowel obstructions by Bastug et al. in 1991 for a patient with an obstruction secondary to a solitary adhesive band [9]. Many subsequent studies have been conducted on the successful use of minimally invasive surgery for small bowel obstructions. However, no prospective randomized trials comparing laparoscopic to open adhesiolysis exist to date, and certainly no consensus statement exists on the gold standard approach to small bowel obstruction. Despite this paucity of data, according to a large review of the American College of Surgeons National Surgical Quality Improvement Program data, a trend exists nationally toward an increase in the adoption of laparoscopic adhesiolysis by 1.6% per year, increasing from 17.2% in 2006 to 28.7% in 2013 [2]. With this increasing trend, high-volume centers have shorter postoperative length of stay with a minimally invasive approach, even when adjusted for case complexity [19]. Despite the increasing trend and acceptance of minimally invasive adhesiolysis as a safe and feasible approach, the use of the minimally invasive techniques for operative management of small bowel obstruction has been demonstrated to be underutilized [21].

## Crohn's Disease

Minimally invasive surgery has also been explored in the setting of Crohn's disease involving the small intestine. Despite the proven benefits of laparoscopy compared to open surgery in small and large intestinal surgery, surgeons have been apprehensive to apply these techniques to patients with Crohn's disease due to the disease process itself. Some of these reservations stem from the concern of inability to identify all occult segments of diseased bowel; lack of tactile sense to identify proximal strictures; possibility of reduced immune response induced by laparoscopy, resulting in earlier recurrence; and the difficulty of operating on friable, inflamed bowel and mesentery, which can possibly be complicated further by dense adhesions, fistulas, and abscesses. These concerns of applying minimally invasive techniques to the surgical management of Crohn's disease were the premise of a Cochrane review in 2011, comparing the use of laparoscopic surgery to open surgery for Crohn's disease and addressing the safety and feasibility of the laparoscopic approach to this disease process. The review focused on the most common procedures performed for Crohn's disease of the small bowel, including ileocecectomy, small bowel resection, and stricturoplasty. Two randomized control trials were included in the review, demonstrating laparoscopic surgery to be associated with a reduced number of wound infections and decreased reoperation rates for non-disease-related complications, but these differences were not statistically significant. Furthermore, no statistically significant difference was noted in the compared outcomes between laparoscopic and open surgery for Crohn's disease. Ultimately, the authors concluded that the minimally invasive approach to small bowel Crohn's disease was safe with no significant difference in perioperative outcomes or long-term reoperation rates, both disease and non-disease related [5].

## Small Bowel Tumors

Minimally invasive surgery has been proven to be comparable to open surgery by oncologic standards for many malignancies, including pancreas, gastric, and colorectal cancer. Conversely, the data comparing minimally invasive surgery to open surgery for neoplasms of the small intestinal tract are scarce [22–25]. Several studies have demonstrated laparoscopic surgery to be safe and oncologically equivalent to open surgery in the setting of small bowel GIST and small bowel NET, particularly when an R0 resection (microscopically and macroscopically negative margins) is achieved for both malignancies and an adequate lymphadenectomy is achieved in the setting of small bowel NET [14, 15, 26, 27].

In the setting of small bowel NET, thorough exploration of the entire small bowel either laparoscopically or open from the ligament of Treitz to ileocecal valve is essential in ensuring no lesions are missed. Controversy still exits for the role of laparoscopy in small bowel NET given the often small size of the primary small bowel NET and the known possibility of having multiple small bowel NET. For smaller NET of the small intestine, endoscopy can assist in identifying the lesion and its location [27]. A few studies have been performed specifically examining the role of laparoscopy for small intestine carcinoid. The only retrospective study on the topic was reported by Reissman et al. in 2014, demonstrating 20 patients with midgut carcinoid tumor who underwent laparoscopic resection en bloc with resection of the corresponding mesenteric root mass suffered no major morbidities. Two patients (10%) experienced minor morbidity, consisting of a wound infection and prolonged ileus. None of the 20 patients required conversion to an open operation. This study demonstrated laparoscopic resection of midgut carcinoid tumors to be a safe, feasible, and oncologically sound surgical approach to these tumors [28]. However, additional studies are necessary prior to accepting a minimally invasive approach to small bowel NET as the gold standard.

As for appendiceal carcinoids, these tumors are often resected incidentally when surgery is performed for presumed appendicitis or during a gynecologic procedure, both of which are commonly performed via a laparoscopic technique. As with primary midgut carcinoid, laparoscopic resection of appendiceal carcinoid tumor is not currently the gold standard; however, it is widely accepted by most surgeons [27]. More extensive surgery, such as a right hemicolectomy, may be necessary based on the size of the lesion, proximity to the base of the appendix, nodal involvement, and other factors. Minimally invasive approaches to appendiceal tumors will be covered later in this chapter as well.

Case reports and series have also been published supporting minimally invasive surgical approaches to adenocarcinoma of the small bowel as well as metastatic lesions to the small bowel; however, further studies are necessary to better define this indication [15, 29, 30].

## Meckel's Diverticulum

Meckel's diverticulum, resulting from an obliteration defect of the omphalomesenteric duct, is one of the most common gastrointestinal malformations, present in 2–4% of the population [31, 32]. Symptomatic Meckel's diverticulum generally presents as a gastrointestinal bleed due to ectopic gastric mucosa in younger patients and more acutely in the adult population, complicated by inflammation, obstruction, perforation, ulceration, and hemorrhage. The treatment for Meckel's diverticulum is surgical, typically consisting of a diverticulectomy, wedge resection of the diverticulum containing the heterotopic mucosa (usually gastric or pancreatic), or segmental resection of the small intestine and primary anastomosis. Traditionally, these procedures have been performed with a laparotomy incision; however, laparoscopy is being utilized more often. A meta-analysis reporting on 35 cases by Abul Hosn et al. and several other studies and case reports have demonstrated safety and efficacy with a laparoscopic approach to this disease process, even in the pediatric setting [31, 33, 34]. Nonetheless, more formal studies have not been conducted to form a consensus statement on the best surgical approach to Meckel's diverticulum.

## Appendicitis

Over the past 15 years, laparoscopic appendectomy has been accepted as improving diagnostic accuracy and decreasing wound infection rates over open appendectomy. According to the Society of American Gastrointestinal and Endoscopic Surgeons (SAGES) guidelines, laparoscopic appendectomy is safe and effective for treating uncomplicated appendicitis and may be used as an alternative to an open appendectomy. Despite longer operative times laparoscopically, several randomized control studies demonstrated laparoscopic appendectomy to be associated with shorter hospital stay and possibly quicker return to work, supporting laparoscopic appendectomy as an alternative to open appendectomy in the SAGES guidelines. Furthermore, meta-analyses demonstrated open appendectomy resulted in increased pain, longer length of stay, and increased wound infection rate compared to laparoscopic appendectomy.

For patients with complicated or perforated appendicitis, no randomized controlled trials have been performed comparing open appendectomy to laparoscopic appendectomy. However, multiple studies have verified that the laparoscopic technique is feasible and safe in the setting of perforated appendicitis. Many of the reports had variable complication rates between the two approaches but generally demonstrated a lower wound infection rate, shorter length of stay, and decreased morbidity and mortality for laparoscopic appendectomy compared to open appendectomy [35].

## Appendiceal Neoplasms

Appendiceal neoplasms encompass a wide range of disease processes, ranging from benign to malignant and including leiomyomas, neuromas, lipomas, carcinoids, mucinous neoplasms, and adenocarcinoma. The role of surgery varies based on the underlying disease process and the histology of the neoplasm. While there is no consensus statement for the minimally invasive approach to appendiceal neoplasms, some retrospective studies have demonstrated a minimally invasive approach resulted in slightly higher rates of margin positivity but had similar 5-year survival rates compared to open appendectomy [36].

Appendiceal carcinoid tumors, a specific type of appendiceal neoplasm, can be managed with either an appendectomy or a right hemicolectomy, based on the size of the lesion, proximity to the base of the appendix, nodal involvement, and other such factors. Since many of these tumors present as presumed appendicitis, appendiceal carcinoid tumors are often resected with a laparoscopic appendectomy prior to diagnosis [37]. Many retrospective reviews, including the review by Park et al., demonstrate the safety and feasibility of a minimally invasive approach for appendiceal tumors. This is particularly notable in the setting of appendiceal mucinous neoplasms given the potential for mucinous spillage and increased risk of pseudomyxoma peritonea for a ruptured lesion [38]. As for appendiceal adenocarcinoma, these neoplasms typically behave as colon cancers, requiring a right hemicolectomy for adequate lymph node harvest to appropriately stage the tumor. In a study of 94 patients with primary appendiceal adenocarcinoma, 12 patients (38%) were upstaged based upon the final pathology following a right hemicolectomy compared to the pathology following an appendectomy [39]. As in colon cancer, a right hemicolectomy can be performed safely and effectively using a minimally invasively approach.

## Less Common Applications

Minimally invasive techniques have been applied to more complicated surgical processes previously thought to not be amenable to this technique, such as gastrointestinal bleeds [40]. At times, this technique can be aided by the use of double-balloon enteroscopy [41]. The minimally invasive technique has also been utilized successfully in identifying and removing foreign bodies, at times requiring small bowel resection with primary anastomosis [42, 43]. Some case reports have also been published on the laparoscopic approach to gallstone ileus, in which a laparoscopic enterotomy with stone extraction is performed safely [44, 45]. Similarly, only case reports and a small case series consisting of three patients with intussusception were successfully managed with laparoscopic-assisted small bowel resection as reported by Siow and Mahendran [46].

## Robotic Surgery

As seen in other organs, many of the same principles used to manage and treat surgical problems afflicting the small bowel can be applied with a robotic approach to the same disease process. While the robot has improved optics and more precise movements, it lacks the haptic feedback afforded by the laparoscopic and open approach. Although no consensus statement has been currently made regarding the safety, feasibility, and use of robotic surgery for small bowel surgery, many case reports and case series are emerging to suggest robotic surgery as an acceptable alternative to open surgery. As more and more surgeons overcome the learning curve for robotic surgery, studies will need to be performed more formally to assess the safety of this technique in small bowel surgery.

## Limitations and Contraindications of Minimally Invasive Surgery

While not considered contraindications, caution should be taken in the setting of technically challenging situations, such as prior laparotomy, obesity, and adhesions to name a few. The severity of disease can also contribute to a higher rate of conversion from a minimally invasive approach to an open approach, including massively dilated loops of small bowel, enterocutaneous fistula, large inflammatory masses, extensive inflammation, and difficulty safely identifying the anatomy [1, 47]. Other relative contraindications include hypotension, septic shock, and inability to establish pneumoperitoneum. Emergency operations performed laparoscopically have also been associated with higher rates of conversion to an open procedure but are not prohibitive to a minimally invasive approach, which at times can be beneficial to the patient [1, 7]. Experience can also contribute to the surgeon's ability to complete an operation in a minimally invasive fashion [48, 49].

## Postoperative Complications

While generally beneficial to the patient, a minimally invasive approach to small bowel surgery can have several potential complications. Complications have been associated with simply entering the abdomen with either a Veress needle or trocar insertion, including injury to major retroperitoneal vessels and/or bowel, abdominal wall hematoma, wound infection, fascial dehiscence, and herniation. In order to perform an operation utilizing a minimally invasive approach, pneumoperitoneum must be achieved. However, pneumoperitoneum results in its own complications, including respiratory acidosis from the carbon dioxide used to insufflate the abdomen, which then gets absorbed in the body. In addition, pneumoperitoneum results in decreased cardiac output by up to 30% secondary to decreased stroke volume during laparoscopic surgery. There is also an increase in systemic vascular resistance. Consequently, people with poor cardiac performance may require invasive cardiac monitoring to ensure they can tolerate insufflating the abdomen fully [50].

Enterotomies and serosal injuries can occur during minimally invasive surgery for any indication secondary to tearing the bowel during adhesiolysis; manipulating the bowel, especially if the bowel is particularly friable; inadequately visualizing the tips of the instruments; and from thermal injuries secondary to electrocautery [1]. If diagnosed at the time of initial operation, these injuries should be addressed and repaired immediately. Other complications associated with minimally invasive small bowel surgery are inherent to the particular procedure being performed and similar to the complications observed when the procedure is performed with an open approach, such as an anastomotic leak, bleeding, intra-abdominal abscess, wound infection, pulmonary embolism, pneumonia, pleural effusion, atelectasis, acute respiratory distress syndrome, acute coronary syndrome, myocardial infarction, deep vein thrombosis, adhesions requiring re-intervention, and incisional hernias to name of few [51]. The rates of complication vary depending on each of the aforementioned scenarios.

## Conclusions

Minimally invasive surgery is a safe, feasible, and efficacious approach to the management of surgical disease processes of the small intestine. Precluding certain situations where it is contraindicated, a minimally invasive approach to small bowel surgery is recommended in the hands of a skilled surgeon experienced in minimally invasive techniques.

# References

1. Zeni TM, Bemelman WA, Frantzides CT. Chap. 11 Minimally invasive procedures on the small intestine. In: Frantzides CT, Carlson MA, editors. Atlas of minimally invasive surgery. Philadelphia: Saunders Elsevier; 2009. p. 97–101.
2. Pei KY, Asuzu D, Davis KA. Will laparoscopic lysis of adhesions become the standard of care? Evaluating trends and outcomes in laparoscopic management of small-bowel obstruction using the American College of Surgeons National Surgical Quality Improvement Project Database. Surg Endosc. 2017;31(5):2180–6.
3. Guo D, Gong J, Cao L, Wei Y, Guo Z, Zhu W. Laparoscopic surgery can reduce postoperative edema compared with open surgery. Gastroenterol Res Pract. 2016.
4. Switzer NJ, Gill RS, Karmali S. The evolution of the appendectomy: from open to laparoscopic to single incision. Scientifica. 2012:Article ID 895469.
5. Dasari BV, McKay D, Gardiner K. Laparoscopic versus open surgery for small bowel Crohn's disease. Cochrane Database Syst Rev. 2011 Jan 19;1:CD006956.
6. Navez B, Navez J. Laparoscopy in the acute abdomen. Best Pract Res Clin Gastroenterol. 2014;28(1):3–17.
7. Matsevych OY, Koto MZ, Aldous C. Laparoscopic-assisted approach for penetrating abdominal trauma: A solution for multiple bowel injuries. Int J Surg. 2017;44:94–8.
8. Cologne KG, Senagore AJ. Development of minimally invasive colorectal surgery: history, evidence, learning curve, and current adaptation. Advanced techniques in minimally invasive and robotic colorectal surgery. New York: Springer; 2015.
9. Bastug DF, Trammell SW, Boland JP, Mantz EP, Tiley EH. 3rd laparoscopic adhesiolysis for small bowel obstruction. Surg Laparosc Endosc. 1991;1:259–62.
10. Antoniou SA, Antoniou GA, Koch OO, Pointner R, Granderath FA. Is laparoscopic ileocecal resection a safe option for Crohn's disease? Best evidence topic. Int J Surg. 2014;12(5):22–5.
11. Ding Y, Zhou Y, Ji Z, Zhang J, Wang Q. Laparoscopic management of perforated Meckel's diverticulum in adults. Int J Med Sci. 2012;9(3):243–7.
12. Sun Z, Rodriguez J, McMichael J, Walsh RM, Chalikonda S, Rosenthal RJ, Kroh MD, El-Hayek K. Minimally invasive duodenojejunostomy for superior mesenteric artery syndrome: a case series and review of the literature. Surg Endosc. 2015;29(5):1137–44.
13. Tabrizian P, Sweeney RE, Uhr JH, Nguyen SQ, Divino CM. Laparoscopic resection of gastric and small bowel gastrointestinal stromal tumors: 10-year experience at a single center. J Am Coll Surg. 2014;218(3):367–73.
14. Figueiredo MN, Maggiori L, Gaujoux S, Couvelard A, Guedj N, Ruszniewski P, Panis Y. Surgery for small-bowel neuroendocrine tumors: is there any benefit of the laparoscopic approach? Surg Endosc. 2014;28(5):1720–6.
15. Tsui DK, Tang CN, Ha JP, Li MK. Laparoscopic approach for small bowel tumors. Surg Laparosc Endosc Percutan Tech. 2008;18(6):556–60.
16. Hamm JK, Chaudhery SI, Kim RH. Laparoscopic resection of small bowel sarcoma. Surg Laparosc Endosc Percutan Tech. 2013;23(3):e138–40.
17. Abdullah MT, Waqar SH, Zahid MA. Laparoscopy in unexplained abdominal pain: surgeon's perspective. J Ayub Med Coll Abbottabad. 2016;28(3):461–4.
18. Ayloo SM, Masrur MA, Bianco FM, Giulianotti PC. Robotic Roux-en-Y duodenojejunostomy for superior mesenteric artery syndrome: operative technique. J Laparoendosc Adv Surg Tech A. 2011;21(9):841–4.
19. Jean RA, O'Neill KM, Pei KY, Davis KA. Impact of hospital volume on outcomes for laparoscopic adhesiolysis for small bowel obstruction. J Surg Res. 2017;214:23–31.
20. Nagle A, Ujiki M, Denham W, Murayama K. Laparoscopic adhesiolysis for small bowel obstruction. Am J Surg. 2004;187(4):464–70.
21. Daly SC, Popoff AM, Fogg L, Francescatti AB, Myers JA, Millikan KW, Deziel DJ, Luu MB. Minimally invasive technique leads to decreased morbidity and mortality in small bowel

resections compared to an open technique: an ACS-NSQIP identified target for improvement. J Gastrointest Surg. 2014;18(6):1171–5. https://doi.org/10.1007/s11605-014-2493-5.
22. Ma Y, Yang Z, Qin H, et al. A meta-analysis of laparoscopy compared with open colorectal resection for colorectal cancer. MedOncol. 2011;28:925–33.
23. Kooby DA, Hawkins WG, Schmidt CM, et al. A multicenter analysis of distal pancreatectomy for adenocarcinoma: Is laparo-scopic resection appropriate? J Am Coll Surg. 2010;210:779–85, 786–777.
24. Mehrabi A, Hafezi M, Arvin J, et al. A systematic review and meta-analysis of laparoscopic versus open distal pancreatectomy for benign and malignant lesions of the pancreas: It's time to randomize. Surgery. 2015;157:45–55.
25. Spolverato G, Kim Y, Ejaz A, et al. A multi-institutional analysis of open versus minimally-invasive surgery for gastric adenocarcinoma: Results of the US gastric cancer collaborative. J Gastrointest Surg. 2014;18:1563–74.
26. Matlok M, Stanek M, Pedziwiatr M, Major P, Kulawik J, Budzynski P. Laparoscopic surgery in the treatment of gastrointestinal stromal tumors. Scand J Surg. 2015;104(3):185–90.
27. Shamiyeh A, Gabriel M. Laparoscopic resection of gastrointestinal neuroendocrine tumors with special contribution of radionuclide imaging. World J Gastroenterol. 2014;20(42):15608–15.
28. Reissman P, Shmailov S, Grozinsky-Glasberg S, Gross DJ. Laparoscopic resection of primary midgut carcinoid tumors. Surg Endosc. 2013;27(10):3678–82.
29. Napolitano L, Waku M, De Nicola P, Di Bartolomeo N, Aceto L, Innocenti P. Surgical laparo-scopic therapy of small bowel tumors: review of the literature and report of two cases. G Chir. 2004;25(6–7):235–7.
30. Felsher J, Brodsky J, Brody F. Laparoscopic small bowel resection of metastatic pulmonary carcinosarcoma. J Laparoendosc Adv Surg Tech A. 2003;13(6):397–400.
31. Hosn MA, Lakis M, Faraj W, Khoury G, Diba S. Laparoscopic approach to symptomatic Meckel diverticulum in adults. JSLS. 2014;18(4). pii: e2014.00349.
32. Papparella A, Nino F, Noviello C, Marte A, Parmeggiani P, Martino A, Cobellis G. Laparoscopic approach to Meckel's diverticulum. World J Gastroenterol. 2014;20(25): 8173–8. https://doi.org/10.3748/wjg.v20.i25.8173.
33. Chan KW, Lee KH, Mou JW, Cheung ST, Tam YH. Laparoscopic management of complicated Meckel's diverticulum in children: a 10-year review. Surg Endosc. 2008;22(6):1509–12.
34. Alemayehu H, Stringel G, Lo IJ, Golden J, Pandya S, McBride W, Muensterer O. Laparoscopy and complicated Meckel diverticulum in children. JSLS. 2014;18(3):e2014.00015.
35. Guidelines for Laparoscopic Appendectomy. © 2017 Society of American Gastrointestinal and Endoscopic Surgeon. sages.org/publications/guidelines/guidelines-for-laparoscopic-appendectomy/
36. Bucher P, Mathe Z, Demirag A, Morel PH. Appendix tumors in the era of laparoscopic appen-dectomy. Surg Endosc. 2004;18(7):1063–6.
37. Grozinsky-Glasberg S, Alexandraki KI, Barak D, Doviner V, Reissman P, Kaltsas GA, Gross DJ. Current size criteria for the management of neuroendocrine tumors of the appendix: are they valid? Clinical experience and review of the literature. Neuroendocrinology. 2013;98(1):31–7.
38. Park KJ, Choi HJ, Kim SH. Laparoscopic approach to mucocele of appendiceal mucinous cystadenoma: feasibility and short-term outcomes in 24 consecutive cases. Surg Endosc. 2015;29(11):3179–83.
39. Nitecki SS, Wolff BG, Schlinkert R, Sarr MG. The natural history of surgically treated primary adenocarcinoma of the appendix. Ann Surg. 1994;219:51–7.
40. Ertem M, Ozben V, Ozveri E, Yilmaz S. Application of laparoscopy in the management of obscure gastrointestinal bleeding. Surg Laparosc Endosc Percutan Tech. 2010;20(2):89–92.
41. Masrur M, Daskalaki D, Vannucchi A, Vannemreddy SN, Gonzalez-Ciccarelli LF, Brown R, Giulianotti PC. Minimally invasive treatment of difficult bleeding lesions of the small bowel. Minerva Chir. 2016;71(5):293–9.

42. Dural AC, Çelik MF, Yiğitbaş H, Akarsu C, Doğan M, Alış H. Laparoscopic resection and intracorporeal anastomosis of perforated small bowel caused by fish bone ingestion. Ulus Travma Acil Cerrahi Derg. 2016;22(6):572–4.
43. Wichmann MW, Hüttl TP, Billing A, Jauch KW. Laparoscopic management of a small bowel perforation caused by a toothpick. Surg Endosc. 2004;18(4):717–8.
44. Coisy M, Bourgouin S, Chevance J, Balandraud P. Laparoscopic management of gallstone ileus. J Gastrointest Surg. 2016;20(2):476–8.
45. Bircan HY, Koc B, Ozcelik U, Kemik O, Demirag A. Laparoscopic treatment of gallstone ileus. Clin Med Insights Case Rep. 2014;7:75–7.
46. Siow SL, Mahendran HA. A case series of adult intussusception managed laparoscopically. Surg Laparosc Endosc Percutan Tech. 2014;24(4):327–31.
47. Schmidt CM, Talamini MA, Kaufman HS, Lilliemoe KD, Learn P, Bayless T. Laparoscopic surgery for Crohn's disease: reasons for conversion. Ann Surg. 2001;233(6):733–9.
48. Evans J, Poritz L, MacRae H. Influence of experience on laparoscopic ileocolic resection for Crohn's disease. Dis Colon Rectum. 2002;45(12):1595–600.
49. Rashidi L, Neighorn C, Bastawrous A. Outcome comparisons between high-volume robotic and laparoscopic surgeons in a large healthcare system. Am J Surg. 2017;213(5):901–5.
50. Perugini RA, Callery MP. Complications of laparoscopic surgery. Surgical treatment: evidence-based and problem-oriented. In: Holzheimer RG, Mannick JA, editors. Surgical treatment: evidence-based and problem-oriented. Munich: Zuckschwerdt; 2001.
51. Cirocchi R, Abraha I, Farinella E, Montedori A, Sciannameo F. Laparoscopic versus open surgery in small bowel obstruction. Cochrane Database Syst Rev. 2010;2:CD007511.

# Chapter 10
# Malignant: Polyps and Cancer

Alessio Pigazzi and Matthew T. Brady

## Introduction

Colon and rectal cancer together make up the second leading cause of cancer-related deaths in the United States in both men and women combined. The National Cancer Institute estimated 135,430 new cases of colon and rectal cancer were diagnosed in 2017, accounting for 8% of all cancer diagnoses. Current estimates place the prevalence of colorectal cancer at 1.3 million people within the United States currently. Additionally there were an estimated 50,260 deaths as a result of colon and rectal cancer, accounting for 8.4% of all cancer-related deaths.

Survival in colon and rectal cancer is stage dependent. The tumor, node, metastasis (TNM) model of staging is very useful in predicting survival outcome among patients being treated for colon and rectal cancer. These measures are assessed with a variety of modalities. Patients will also typically undergo colonoscopic evaluation to estimate the tumor location in conjunction with tattooing of the tumor to aid during operative resection. For rectal cancer, assessment of tumor and nodal stage is performed with pelvic magnetic resonance imaging (MRI) or endorectal ultrasound (EUS). Computed tomography (CT) is used in both colon and rectal cancer to assess for distant solid tumor metastases commonly in the liver and lung.

Minimally invasive surgery is a term that encompasses numerous surgical techniques including endoscopy, laparoscopy, and robotic-assisted surgery. When

A. Pigazzi, MD, PhD · M. T. Brady, MD (✉)
Department of Surgery, Division of Colon and Rectal Surgery, University of California Irvine Medical Center, Orange, CA, USA
e-mail: apigazzi@uci.edu; mtbrady@uci.edu

© Springer Nature Switzerland AG 2019
C. Rezac, K. Donohue (eds.), *The Internist's Guide to Minimally Invasive Gastrointestinal Surgery*, Clinical Gastroenterology,
https://doi.org/10.1007/978-3-319-96631-1_10

applied to surgery of the colon and rectum for malignant disease, these techniques share a common goal of achieving the same oncologic results for patients as open surgery while offering improved postoperative recovery and patient satisfaction.

Minimally invasive approaches to surgery for colon and rectal cancer have been demonstrated to be safe when compared to open approaches and offer numerous benefits to the patient [8, 14, 15, 18]. Postoperative outcomes such as surgical site infection, postoperative incisional hernia rate, inpatient hospital length of stay, and postoperative narcotic pain medication usage have all been shown to improve when using a minimally invasive technique [2, 11]. It is helpful to understand what minimally invasive surgery options are available for the treatment of colon and rectal cancer to adequately care for patients presenting with these malignant diseases. Additionally, knowledge of these procedures can help guide referrals for patients seeking specialty care.

## Minimally Invasive Approaches to Colon Cancer

The principles of surgery for colon cancer remain the same regardless of whether approaching the resection through an open or minimally invasive technique. These principles are focused on removal of the primary tumor as well as performing an adequate lymphadenectomy. The National Comprehensive Cancer Network has provided recommendations to guide these principles which include having a minimum of 12 lymph nodes within the resected specimen [4]. Generally, 5 cm proximal and distal resection margins are recommended to help achieve the necessary lymphadenectomy and ensure negative margins. Additionally it is recommended to ligate the primary vascular pedicle of the affected colon at its origin [23]. The concept of a complete mesocolic excision (CME) has been adopted for its improved disease-free survival in patients with colon cancer [5]. This technique involved high ligation of the vascular pedicle to the affected colon and dissection of the embryologic planes between the mesocolon and retroperitoneum. This approach aims to yield a complete lymph node excision. These planes can be very well visualized laparoscopically which aids in complete mesocolic excision at the time of surgery.

As stated previously, minimally invasive surgical approaches have resulted in similar cancer-related outcomes when compared to open resections in multiple prospective randomized trials throughout the world [11, 14, 26]. When compared with open surgery, no differences are seen in number of lymph nodes examined or resection margins. More importantly, no differences in recurrence, disease-free survival, or overall survival have been noted [11]. Improved short-term patient outcomes are seen when a minimally invasive approach is employed. Postoperative length of stay is decreased in patients undergoing laparoscopic colon resection (5 vs. 6 days), as is parenteral narcotic pain medication usage (3 vs. 4 days) [11]. Additionally, incisional hernia and postoperative adhesion formation rates are also minimized when compared with open technique [7]. These improvements can have lasting outcome in a patient's quality of life after surgery and are important considerations in choosing an operative approach.

Minimally invasive operations for colon cancer can be done totally laparoscopically, as is the author's preference, robotically, or with a hand-assisted laparoscopic surgery (HALS) technique in which a specialized gel port is used to allow the surgeon to place a hand in the abdomen during laparoscopy. Advocates for hand-assisted surgery state, it offers the ability to handle tissue similar to open surgery while achieving similar benefits of smaller incisions and improved recovery compared with open techniques. Drawbacks of HALS compared with total laparoscopic techniques are that incision sites are larger, postoperative bowel function recovery is slower, and increased length of stay, compared with total laparoscopic technique, has been reported [20].

The most common approaches for minimally invasive colon resections are described as medial-to-lateral and lateral-to-medical dissections. Each of these approaches aims to dissect the mesocolon in its entirety off the retroperitoneum to perform a CME. A medial-to-lateral dissection involves first elevating the mesocolon of the colon off the retroperitoneum prior to releasing the lateral attachments of the colon at the white line of Toldt. This is performed by placing the mesentery of the colon on stretch, and identifying the vascular pedicle of interest begins this process. Once identified, the peritoneum lying posterior to this pedicle is incised in an axis parallel to the vessel, and the embryologic fusion plane between the mesocolon and the retroperitoneum is developed. This plane is developed using a combination of electrocautery, sharp, and blunt dissection. In laparoscopy, the pressure of the abdominal insufflation causes the carbon dioxide to dissect into the avascular plane between the mesocolon and retroperitoneum, aiding in the dissection. During this dissection it is critical to ensure the retroperitoneal structures such as the ureters, gonadal vessels, and duodenum remain posterior to the plane of dissection as they can easily be elevated with the colon if care is not taken. The lateral-to-medial approach more mirrors the open technique. In this approach the lateral attachments to the colon at the white line of Toldt are incised, and the colon is elevated off the retroperitoneum medially. In this technique the colon is typically freed from its retroperitoneal attachments prior to ligation or division of the vascular pedicle.

The approach and technique used is largely dependent on both surgeon and patient factors. Surgeon's training experience, expertise, and preference, as well as patient factors, typically dictate which technique is employed.

## *Minimally Invasive Approaches to Rectal Cancer*

Despite similarities in pathogenesis, the surgical management of rectal cancer has distinct features which differentiate it from colon cancer. The preoperative determination of both the T and N stage of the rectal cancer, as well as its distance from the anorectal sphincter complex, is imperative for the proper care of these patients given the availability of neoadjuvant chemoradiation in appropriate cases. Minimally invasive surgical approaches to rectal tumors include transanal endoscopic surgery (TES), laparoscopic- and robotic-assisted low anterior resection (LAR), and laparoscopic- and robotic-assisted abdominoperineal resection (APR). The decision of which surgical approach to use when caring for a patient with rectal cancer is dependent on both tumor-related and patient factors. The choice of surgery needs to balance the likelihood of a curative resection with the patient's ability to tolerate the operation, the feasibility of sphincter preservation, and postoperative alteration of bowel function.

## Transanal Endoscopic Surgery

Rectal polyps which are unresectable, as well as T1 cancers of the rectum, can be resected using a transanal approach. The NCCN guidelines provide recommendations for physical characteristics of a rectal tumor that make it appropriate for a transanal excision which include a mobile, nonfixed, T1 tumor, less than 3 cm in dimension and within 8 cm of the anal verge [12]. These parameters likely reflect the appropriateness for an excision based on accessibility of the lesions. Modern minimally invasive transanal techniques have made the resection of higher and larger lesions feasible by allowing closure of the remaining defect in the rectal wall using absorbable sutures. With this technique even full-thickness rectal wall excisions of the proximal rectum that enter the peritoneal cavity can be successfully closed with low morbidity [13].

Transanal endoscopic surgery (TES) has its origin in the 1980s when the platform of transanal endoscopic microsurgery (TEM) was developed [10]. This platform involved a rectoscope with a sealed faceplate of multi-access ports which permitted surgeons to work with laparoscopic instruments while insufflating the rectum with carbon dioxide to create a working space. The unit had high upfront costs as well as a steep learning curve and as such adoption was limited though has grown more recently. In 2010, transanal minimally invasive surgery (TAMIS) was described. This technique is very similar to TEM, but instead of a dedicated rectoscope, it uses a nonrigid port designed for single-incision laparoscopic surgery [3]. This allows surgeons to perform TES and achieve similar outcomes to TEM but with decreased upfront costs associated with TEM [1, 3]. Overall these techniques are quite similar in their use of a multi-access port and rectal insufflation with carbon dioxide to maintain a working space (Fig. 10.1).

TES is very useful for rectal polyps that cannot be excised in their entirety through traditional endoscopic techniques. TES allows for both mucosal and full-thickness excisions and can allow for improved T staging by providing the pathologist with a full-thickness biopsy unlike what can be provided with a piecemeal resection through a flexible endoscope [28]. The ability to obtain full-thickness excision can help guide decisions to pursue more aggressive surgical approaches in including low anterior resection (LAR) or abdominoperineal resection (APR). Compared with conventional transanal excision, TES offers improved quality of excisions with less fragmented specimens (1–6% vs. 24–35%), decreased incidence of positive margins (10–12% vs. 29–50%), and decreased rates of local recurrence (5–6% vs. 27–29%)[19, 21, 22].

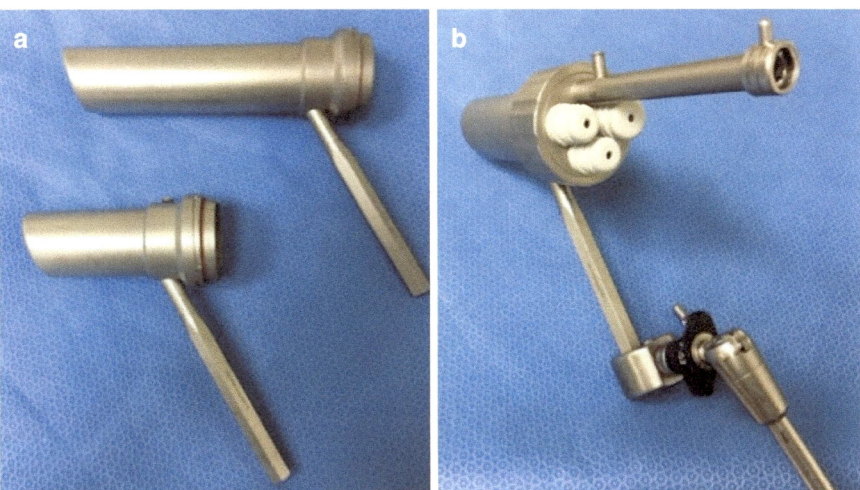

**Fig. 10.1** Transanal Endoscopic Surgery unit produced Karl Storz, Germany. The unit consists of a rigid rectoscope (**a**) which have multiple lengths depending on the distance of the lesion from the anal verge. The unit has a sealed faceplate (**b**) to maintain insufflation within the rectum. Laparoscopic instruments and an endoscopic camera is inserted to perform the transanal resection

Historically, transanal excision (TAE) of rectal tumors has been associated with increased rates of local recurrence compared with proctectomy. A 2015 meta-analysis comparing TAE to proctectomy for resection of T1 N0 rectal adenocarcinoma demonstrated this as well, though a subgroup analysis revealed no difference in local recurrence rates for patients who had undergone TES and proctectomy, showing benefit for the minimally invasive technique over TAE. Considering the decrease in mortality, postoperative complications, and likelihood of stoma creation associated with transanal excision when compared with proctectomy, the authors in this study favored TES for T1 N0 rectal cancer.

## Laparoscopic and Robotic Approaches to Rectal Cancer

Low anterior resections of the rectum are performed for patients with rectal cancer in whom an oncologic resection can be performed while preserving the anorectal sphincter complex. NCCN guidelines recommend a 4–5 cm distal margin for rectal cancer to ensure an adequate mesorectal excision, though for low tumors which are <5 cm from the anal verge NCCN guidelines state a 1–2 cm margin may be acceptable [12]. In addition to resection margins, the performance of a total mesorectal excision (TME) is imperative for the treatment of rectal cancer. The goal of TME is both removal of the rectal cancer as well as the complete excision of the rectal lymph nodes contained within the thin fascial sheath, the fascia propria, of the mesorectum. This technique, first described in 1982, is the gold standard in surgical treatment of rectal cancer [12, 16]. The accomplishment of these goals is made difficult by the anatomic constraints of the pelvis. Operative exposure within the pelvis can be technically challenging. The bony confines and pelvic geometry, especially in men, can make operative exposure difficult. This can prove to be even more difficult with bulky rectal tumors and radiation changes to the tissue where a large tissue volume is occupying a small space. Adding to the challenge, critical structures such as the autonomic nerves that control bladder and sexual function, the presacral venous plexus, ureters, iliac vessels, the seminal vesicles, and prostate in men and vaginal wall in women all lie intimately close to the planes of dissection. As described earlier in this chapter, laparoscopic and robotic approaches to rectal cancer have been shown to be safe when compared to an open operation [9, 14, 18].

The use of minimally invasive approaches to pelvic surgery can allow for improved visualization for the operative team in these small confines. This visualization helps identify critical structures in the dissection including the autonomic pelvic nerves which control urinary and sexual function. The RObotic versus LAparoscopic Resection for Rectal Cancer (ROLARR) trial is a randomized trial that examined the compared effectiveness of these two techniques. Laparoscopic TME had been quoted to have a 16% conversion rate to open [9]. Robotic TME is thought to reduce this conversion rate. Interestingly the ROLARR trial did not show a difference in conversion rate to open surgery between robotic and laparoscopic techniques, 8.1% vs. 12.2% $p = 0.16$, in the unadjusted rates. Also, there were no differences in secondary endpoints including rates of circumferential margin positivity, intraoperative complications, postoperative complications, 30-day mortality, or urinary or sexual dysfunction. Multiregression analysis did reveal that there was less conversion to open in the robotic group in men, obese patients, and planned low anterior resections as opposed to planned abdominoperineal resections. These subgroups may suggest that more challenging pelvic anatomy may see a benefit from robotic approach. [17].

TME has been shown to decrease rates of postoperative urinary and sexual dysfunction, likely as a result of improved visualization of the autonomic nerves as the course into the pelvis [24, 27]. Robotic TME has also been shown to have a decreased intraoperative blood loss when compared with open TME [6]. Additionally, the use of a robotic approach can decrease surgeon fatigue during low pelvic dissection [25].

# References

1. Albert MR, Atallah SB, Debeche-Adams TC, Izfar S, Larach SW. Transanal minimally invasive surgery (TAMIS) for local excision of benign neoplasms and early-stage rectal cancer: efficacy and outcomes in the first 50 patients. Dis Colon Rectum. 2013;56:301–7.
2. Andersen LP, Klein M, Gogenur I, Rosenberg J. Incisional hernia after open versus laparoscopic sigmoid resection. Surg Endosc. 2008;22:2026–9.

3. Atallah S, Albert M, Larach S. Transanal minimally invasive surgery: a giant leap forward. Surg Endosc. 2010;24:2200–5.
4. Benson AB 3rd, Venook AP, Cederquist L, Chan E, Chen YJ, Cooper HS, Deming D, Engstrom PF, Enzinger PC, Fichera A, Grem JL, Grothey A, Hochster HS, Hoffe S, Hunt S, Kamel A, Kirilcuk N, Krishnamurthi S, Messersmith WA, Mulcahy MF, Murphy JD, Nurkin S, Saltz L, Sharma S, Shibata D, Skibber JM, Sofocleous CT, Stoffel EM, Stotsky-Himelfarb E, Willett CG, Wu CS, Gregory KM, Deborah Freedman-Cass. Colon cancer, version 1.2017, NCCN clinical practice guidelines in oncology. J Natl Compr Canc Netw. 2017;15:370–98.
5. Bertelsen CA, Neuenschwander AU, Jansen JE, Wilhelmsen M, Kirkegaard-Klitbo A, Tenma JR, Bols B, Ingeholm P, Rasmussen LA, Jepsen LV, Iversen ER, Kristensen B, Gogenur I, Danish Colorectal Cancer G. Disease-free survival after complete mesocolic excision compared with conventional colon cancer surgery: a retrospective, population-based study. Lancet Oncol. 2015;16:161–8.
6. Biffi R, Luca F, Pozzi S, Cenciarelli S, Valvo M, Sonzogni A, Radice D, Ghezzi TL. Operative blood loss and use of blood products after full robotic and conventional low anterior resection with total mesorectal excision for treatment of rectal cancer. J Robot Surg. 2011;5:101–7.
7. Biondi A, Grosso G, Mistretta A, Marventano S, Toscano C, Drago F, Gangi S, Basile F. Laparoscopic vs. open approach for colorectal cancer: evolution over time of minimal invasive surgery. BMC Surg. 2013;13(Suppl 2):S12.
8. Bonjer HJ, Deijen CL, Abis GA, Cuesta MA, van der Pas MH, De Lange-De Klerk ES, Lacy AM, Bemelman WA, Andersson J, Angenete E, Rosenberg J, Fuerst A, Haglind E, COLOR II Study Group. A randomized trial of laparoscopic versus open surgery for rectal cancer. N Engl J Med. 2015a;372:1324–32.
9. Bonjer HJ, Deijen CL, Haglind E, COLOR II Study Group. A randomized trial of laparoscopic versus open surgery for rectal cancer. N Engl J Med. 2015b;373:194.
10. Buess G, Hutterer F, Theiss J, Bobel M, Isselhard W, Pichlmaier H. A system for a transanal endoscopic rectum operation. Chirurg. 1984;55:677–80.
11. Clinical Outcomes of Surgical Therapy Study Group, Nelson H, Sargent DJ, Wieand HS, Fleshman J, Anvari M, Stryker SJ, Beart RW Jr, Hellinger M, Flanagan R Jr, Peters W, Ota D. A comparison of laparoscopically assisted and open colectomy for colon cancer. N Engl J Med. 2004;350:2050–9.
12. Engstrom PF, Arnoletti JP, Benson AB 3rd, Chen YJ, Choti MA, Cooper HS, Covey A, Dilawari RA, Early DS, Enzinger PC, Fakih MG, Fleshman J Jr, Fuchs C, Grem JL, Kiel K, Knol JA, Leong LA, Lin E, Mulcahy MF, Rao S, Ryan DP, Saltz L, Shibata D, Skibber JM, Sofocleous C, Thomas J, Venook AP, Willett C, National Comprehensive Cancer Network. NCCN clinical practice guidelines in oncology: rectal cancer. J Natl Compr Canc Netw. 2009;7:838–81.
13. Gavagan JA, Whiteford MH, Swanstrom LL. Full-thickness intraperitoneal excision by transanal endoscopic microsurgery does not increase short-term complications. Am J Surg. 2004;187:630–4.
14. Green BL, Marshall HC, Collinson F, Quirke P, Guillou P, Jayne DG, Brown JM. Long-term follow-up of the Medical Research Council CLASICC trial of conventional versus laparoscopically assisted resection in colorectal cancer. Br J Surg. 2013;100:75–82.
15. Guillou PJ, Quirke P, Thorpe H, Walker J, Jayne DG, Smith AM, Heath RM, Brown JM, MRC CLASICC Trial Group. Short-term endpoints of conventional versus laparoscopic-assisted surgery in patients with colorectal cancer (MRC CLASICC trial): multicentre, randomised controlled trial. Lancet. 2005;365:1718–26.
16. Heald RJ, Husband EM, Ryall RD. The mesorectum in rectal cancer surgery – the clue to pelvic recurrence? Br J Surg. 1982;69:613–6.
17. Jayne D, Pigazzi A, Marshall H, Croft J, Corrigan N, Copeland J, Quirke P, West N, Rautio T, Thmoassen N, Tilney H, Gudgeon M, Bianchi PP, Edlin R, Hulm C, Brown J. Effect of robotic-assisted vs conventional laparoscopic surgery on risk of conversion to open laparotomy among patients undergoing resection for rectal cancer: the ROLARR randomized clinical trial. JAMA. 2017;318(16):1569–80.

18. Kang SB, Park JW, Jeong SY, Nam BH, Choi HS, Kim DW, Lim SB, Lee TG, Kim DY, Kim JS, Chang HJ, Lee HS, Kim SY, Jung KH, Hong YS, Kim JH, Sohn DK, Kim DH, Oh JH. Open versus laparoscopic surgery for mid or low rectal cancer after neoadjuvant chemoradiotherapy (COREAN trial): short-term outcomes of an open-label randomised controlled trial. Lancet Oncol. 2010;11:637–45.
19. Kidane B, Chadi SA, Kanters S, Colquhoun PH, Ott MC. Local resection compared with radical resection in the treatment of T1N0M0 rectal adenocarcinoma: a systematic review and meta-analysis. Dis Colon Rectum. 2015;58:122–40.
20. Meshikhes AW. Controversy of hand-assisted laparoscopic colorectal surgery. World J Gastroenterol. 2010;16:5662–8.
21. Middleton PF, Sutherland LM, Maddern GJ. Transanal endoscopic microsurgery: a systematic review. Dis Colon Rectum. 2005;48:270 84.
22. Moore JS, Cataldo PA, Osler T, Hyman NH. Transanal endoscopic microsurgery is more effective than traditional transanal excision for resection of rectal masses. Dis Colon Rectum. 2008;51:1026–30; discussion 1030–1.
23. Mutch MG. The ASCRS textbook of colon and rectal surgery. New York: Springer; 2016.
24. Panteleimonitis S, Ahmed J, Harper M, Parvaiz A. Critical analysis of the literature investigating urogenital function preservation following robotic rectal cancer surgery. World J Gastrointest Surg. 2016;8:744–54.
25. Pigazzi A, Ellenhorn JD, Ballantyne GH, Paz IB. Robotic-assisted laparoscopic low anterior resection with total mesorectal excision for rectal cancer. Surg Endosc. 2006;20:1521–5.
26. Veldkamp R, Kuhry E, Hop WC, Jeekel J, Kazemier G, Bonjer HJ, Haglind E, Pahlman L, Cuesta MA, Msika S, Morino M, Lacy AM, COlon Cancer Laparoscopic or Open Resection Study Group (COLOR). Laparoscopic surgery versus open surgery for colon cancer: short-term outcomes of a randomised trial. Lancet Oncol. 2005;6:477–84.
27. Wang G, Wang Z, Jiang Z, Liu J, Zhao J, Li J. Male urinary and sexual function after robotic pelvic autonomic nerve-preserving surgery for rectal cancer. Int J Med Robot. 2017;13:e1725.
28. Whiteford MH. The ASCRS textbook of colon and rectal surgery. New York: Springer; 2016.

## Suggested Readings

National Cancer Institute. Cancer stat facts: colon and rectum cancer [Online]. National Cancer Institute. Available: https://seer.cancer.gov/statfacts/html/colorect.html. Accessed.
Prevention, C. F. D. C. A. Available: https://www.cdc.gov/cancer/colorectal/index.htm. Accessed.

# Chapter 11
# Benign: Volvulus and Diverticulitis

Michelle Y. Chen and Vincent Obias

## Volvulus

### Introduction

When a loop of intestine twists upon itself and its mesentery, a volvulus occurs, leading to bowel obstruction. Volvulus is currently the third most common cause of large bowel obstruction in the world [1]. If twisting of the mesentery compromises the blood supply to the bowel, ischemic bowel can also develop. Volvulus most frequently occurs in middle-aged and elderly men. Risk factors include patients born with intestinal malrotation or Hirschsprung disease (these patients often experience volvulus early in life), pregnancy, enlarged colon, and abdominal adhesions, such as those secondary to abdominal surgery [2]. Patients who are immobilized, including those who are institutionalized or bedbound, are also at an increased risk [3].

The mechanism causing volvulus involves a distended, heavy segment of bowel that becomes susceptible to torsion around its mesentery. This can be due to chronic constipation or a high-fiber diet [2]. A high-fiber diet leads to colon elongation, a predisposing factor to colonic torsion [1]. A study by Akinkuotu et al. also found correlations between anatomic variations and the risk of developing volvulus – patients with longer and wider mesosigmoid colons are more predisposed to developing sigmoid volvulus than those with shorter and narrower mesosigmoids [4].

M. Y. Chen
School of Medicine, The George Washington University, Washington, DC, USA
e-mail: mychen@gwu.edu

V. Obias (✉)
School of Medicine and Health Sciences, George Washington University,
Washington, DC, USA

© Springer Nature Switzerland AG 2019
C. Rezac, K. Donohue (eds.), *The Internist's Guide to Minimally Invasive Gastrointestinal Surgery*, Clinical Gastroenterology,
https://doi.org/10.1007/978-3-319-96631-1_11

In the sigmoid colon, repeated episodes of volvulus can result in shortening of the mesentery and formation of adhesions that fix the colon into a twisted position [2].

Symptoms of volvulus include bloody stools, fever, pain, and symptoms of bowel obstruction such as vomiting, constipation, and obstipation. In the sigmoid colon, constipation is a more prominent symptom, while patients with cecal volvulus will predominantly experience small bowel obstruction symptoms (such as vomiting) [2].

## Types of Volvulus

In adults between the ages of 30 and 70, the most commonly affected site is the sigmoid colon [3]. The second most common site is the cecum, which also involves the terminal ileum and proximal right colon [1]. In order for a cecal volvulus to occur, the cecum must be mobile to permit twisting or folding of the bowel [5]. There are two types of cecal volvulus depending on the mechanism of formation. The first type occurs with axial rotation of bowel around the mesentery of the terminal ileum, cecum, and proximal right colon, usually in a clockwise direction. The second type, known as a cecal bascule, results from the anterosuperior folding of the cecum. There is no actual rotation of bowel with a cecal bascule; therefore, it is less likely to lead to vascular compromise and bowel ischemia. Cecal bascule is also less common than a rotational volvulus and more often occurs in young females [1]. Figure 11.1 shows the abdominal radiograph of a patient with a cecal bascule.

Since both the inflow and the outflow of the affected segment are obstructed, a volvulus is said to be a closed-loop obstruction [3]. This can lead to ischemic bowel, where the segment of the bowel becomes necrotic and acidotic, ultimately leading to bowel wall death. This is a surgical emergency, requiring prompt untwisting of the affected portion of the bowel and restoration of vascular supply [2].

## Diagnosis and Evaluation

Upon evaluation, patients with volvulus appear acutely ill and will report some, if not all, of the symptoms listed above [2]. Additionally, in patients with cecal volvulus, there may be a history of "mobile cecum syndrome," where the patient will report experiencing symptoms intermittently, as the volvulus spontaneously resolves and recurs [1]. On physical exam, in addition to abdominal tenderness and significant abdominal distension, patients may display peritoneal signs and bleeding per rectum [2]. Other signs of intestinal obstruction are also often present, including abdominal tympany and high-pitched bowel sounds. On digital rectum exam, one would find an empty rectum. In some cases, patients can also experience respiratory distress secondary to colonic distension limiting diaphragmatic movement during respiration [3].

**Fig. 11.1** Abdominal radiograph of a cecal bascule

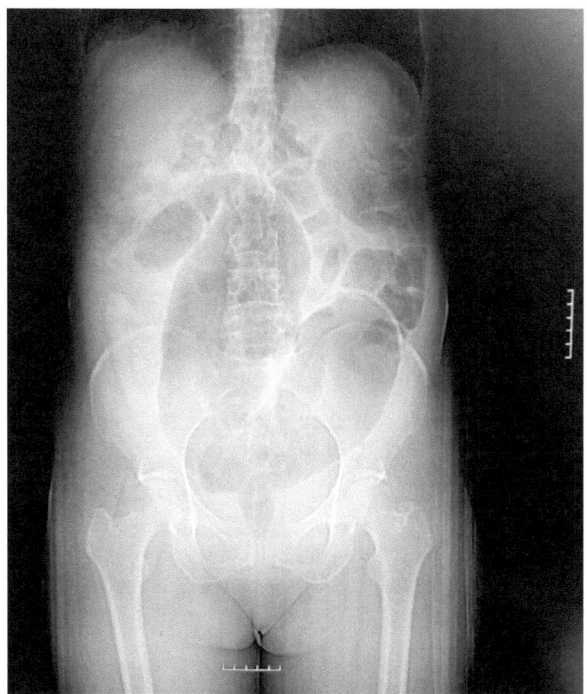

Volvulus is typically diagnosed with imaging, including plain abdominal radiographs, computed tomography (CT), or a gastrointestinal (GI) series. Radiographs alone can be used to diagnose and confirm suspected volvulus [1]. The "coffee bean" sign showing a distended closed loop of colon filled with air, as depicted by Fig. 11.2, is pathognomonic. Barium enema can also be used for evaluation, showing a "bird's beak" at the site where the bowels have twisted [3]. A barium enema can increase the diagnostic accuracy of a radiograph up to 100% [1]. It can also be therapeutic. Barium should be substituted with gastrografin, however, when there is suspicion of bowel perforation. A CT scan is recommended to confirm the diagnosis and to rule out other causes of bowel obstruction, such as carcinoma or polyps [3]. CT usually shows a "whirl" appearance of the mesentery and a distended loop of bowel with air-fluid levels, surrounded by strands of fat and soft tissue [1]. On CT, it is also important to look for free air that would indicate a bowel perforation [3].

## Approaches to Treatment

The initial treatment for sigmoid volvulus involves nonsurgical decompression and detorsion. Seventy to eighty percent of cases of sigmoid volvulus can be successfully decompressed; however, it is less effective in cecal volvulus. Decompression and detorsion can be accomplished with a barium enema, flexible sigmoidoscopy,

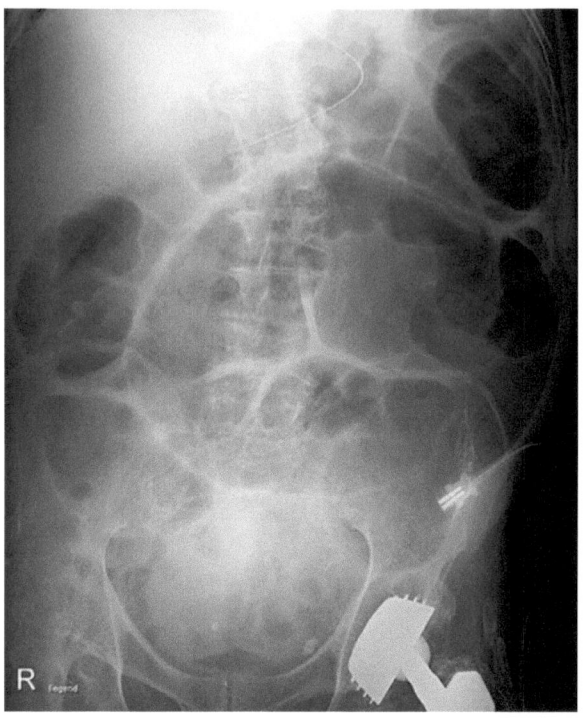

**Fig. 11.2** Coffee bean sign. (From Scharl and Biedermann [6])

colonoscopy, or rigid proctoscopy [1]. Upon endoscopic visualization, if the bowel mucosa looks normal and healthy, a rectal tube is placed for decompression of the bowels [3]. Successful decompression is indicated by the passing of gas and stool [1]. A study conducted by Iida et al. examined endoscopic detorsion in 30 cases of sigmoid volvulus at a single center. The success rate was found to be 62%. Forty-six percent of patients experienced recurrence, and thirty-eight percent of patients required emergency surgery. The factors found to predict successful endoscopic detorsion were the absence of abdominal tenderness, the use of laxatives, and a positive open abdominal surgery history. Although this was a small study, its results are consistent with those of previous reports studying endoscopic detorsion. In general, studies have found the success rate of endoscopic detorsion to range from 55% to 90%; however, given that the rate of recurrence ranges from 35% to 85%, detorsion and decompression are rarely the definitive treatment and is only used as a temporizing measure. Surgery is recommended as the ultimate treatment option, after a patient is medically stabilized, to prevent recurrence [7].

After decompression, the patient should be medically treated to correct any electrolyte, renal, pulmonary, and/or cardiac abnormalities. Once the patient is deemed to be medically stable, elective surgical treatment should be pursued as there is a high rate of recurrence. The recommended time between decompression and surgery is between 48 and 72 h, as this allows for interventions to optimize the patient's health and reduce surgical risk [3]. This will also permit patients to undergo adequate bowel preparation for surgery. Before patients are taken to the operating room, a colonoscopy should be performed to rule out malignancy and other pathologies. However, patients who are acutely septic or febrile, those with leukocytosis, signs of peritonitis, or gangrenous or ischemic bowel visualized upon endoscopy, should undergo immediate colectomy and exploration. These patients should be prepared for surgery with resuscitation, broad-spectrum antibiotics, and nothing-by-mouth protocol. No further diagnostic tests or imaging should be performed. Colonoscopy is not recommended for patients with cecal volvulus; these patients should go directly to surgery [1].

In patients undergoing surgical exploration, a midline incision is performed. The volvulus is identified and the bowel is assessed for viability. If the surgeon determines that the bowel is healthy enough to be salvaged and the patient's overall physiologic status allows for it, the bowel is reduced, and a rectal or cecostomy tube is placed to prevent recurrence. Otherwise, the affected bowel segment should be resected [1]. Elective surgeries after successful decompression are commonly performed through minimally invasive techniques. These include laparoscopy and robotic surgery.

With a colectomy, patients can either receive a primary anastomosis or an end colostomy. A primary anastomosis is performed in most elective cases; however, the final decision is dependent on patient factors, including each patient's nutritional status, comorbidities, and hemodynamic status as well as the adequacy of the blood supply to the bowels, the presence of peritonitis, and the amount of tension exhibited on the bowel by the volvulus. If it is determined that the patient is not a candidate for a primary anastomosis, a Hartmann procedure is performed, creating an end colostomy [1].

In cases of cecal volvulus with normal bowels, a cecopexy can be performed, where the cecum is returned to its original position and sutured into place [2]. This eliminates the prerequisite of a mobile cecum for volvulus to occur. In patients who receive a cecopexy, however, there is a 28% recurrence rate [5]. Most surgeons would do a right hemicolectomy if the patient is stable to reduce recurrence rates. If the bowel is necrotic, a cecopexy is avoided, and a right hemicolectomy with an ileostomy or colostomy is performed to remove the affected segment of bowel and to eliminate the possibility of recurrence [2].

## *Complications*

Volvulus can be complicated by bowel gangrene and necrosis, bowel perforation with peritonitis, and recurrence [2]. The presence of bowel gangrene has been shown to be a prognostic factor. While the average mortality of volvulus is approximately 10%, patients with bowel necrosis experience a mortality of up to 80% [5]. Mortality and morbidity is also high in cases of delayed diagnosis and treatment [2]. Emergent surgical treatment is associated with significant morbidity and mortality, including gangrenous bowel. In patients who only undergo detorsion without surgical resection of the bowel, there is a high risk of recurrence (up to 18%) [5].

# Diverticulitis

## Introduction

Diverticulosis is the presence of outpouchings of the colonic wall, known as diverticula, without inflammation or infection. The majority of diverticula are false, involving only the mucosa and muscularis mucosa, and occur in the sigmoid colon. Diverticula are thought to result from high intraluminal pressure secondary to a lack of dietary fiber, causing high wall tension as stool is propulsed through the colon. The high intraluminal pressure on the colonic wall causes weakening of the bowel wall resulting in pulsion diverticula as the mucosa herniates through the muscularis [8]. Diverticulosis is remarkably prevalent in the United States, affecting approximately 5–10% of people over age 45 and 80% of those over age 85. It is also the most common cause of lower GI bleeding [9]. Risk factors for diverticulosis include factors that contribute to increased intraluminal pressure, including chronic constipation, low fiber intake, increasing age, obesity, and lack of physical activity. Genetic susceptibility also contributes, as monozygotic twins have been shown to be twice as likely to develop diverticulosis compared to dizygotic twins [9].

Diverticulitis refers to the inflammation and infection of diverticula [8]. It results from obstruction of diverticula by a fecalith, leading to diverticular microperforation resulting in colonic wall swelling or macroperforation resulting in involvement of pericolic tissues [9]. It occurs in 10–25% of patients with diverticulosis. It can be categorized as uncomplicated and complicated, which differ in presentation, diagnostic findings, and treatment [8].

## Diagnosis and Evaluation

Patients with uncomplicated diverticulitis most commonly present with acute-onset lower abdominal pain, often in the left lower quadrant (the sigmoid colon is most commonly affected), fever, anorexia, constipation, and/or diarrhea. Initial laboratory tests include a complete blood count as leukocytosis is common feature of diverticulitis. A basic metabolic panel should be obtained to evaluate for any electrolyte abnormalities, especially in patients with decreased oral intake and renal dysfunction. Other tests often obtained include a urinalysis to rule out urinary tract infections, a beta-hCG in women of childbearing age to exclude pregnancy, and a fecal occult blood test to evaluate for GI bleeding [9].

Complicated diverticulitis refers to diverticulitis with abscess formation, >4 cm phlegmon, stricture, perforation, large bowel obstruction (LBO), peritonitis, or fistula formation, including coloenteric, colovesical, and colovaginal fistulas [8]. Clinical presentation varies depending on the complication, ranging from sepsis secondary to peritonitis to emesis, bloating, and constipation or obstipation due to an LBO. Complicated diverticulitis is staged by the Hinchey classification. The Hinchey classification system describes the severity of complicated diverticulitis and is useful in determining approaches to treatment [8].

Hinchey I: with a local (paracolonic) abscess
Hinchey II: with a pelvic or retroperitoneal abscess
Hinchey III: with purulent peritonitis
Hinchey IV: with fecal peritonitis

Imaging studies are not necessary in patients with mild diverticulitis, but they are often obtained in the diagnostic and evaluation process. When diverticular perforation is suspected, an abdominal radiograph is helpful by showing free air. CT is the most commonly used imaging modality and the modality of choice for diagnosing diverticulitis, staging the severity of the episode, and visualizing any complications [10]. It is also helpful for ruling out other conditions with similar presentations, including malignancy, ischemic colitis, and other causes of GI tract inflammation, such as inflammatory bowel disease. The most sensitive CT findings for diverticulitis are thickening of the colonic wall and pericolic fat stranding. CT is also useful in evaluating for diverticulitis complications, including abscesses, phlegmon, LBO, and fistulas. The major disadvantage of CT is exposure to ionizing radiation. Alternative imaging modalities should, therefore, be considered in patients who wish to avoid radiation, especially pregnant women. Other imaging studies often used are ultrasonography and magnetic resonance imaging (MRI); however, each of these comes with their own disadvantages. Ultrasonography is inferior to CT in evaluating for free air and the extent of large abscesses. The accuracy of the study is also variable based on operator technique as well as patient factors, such as body habitus – overweight and obese patients with overlying gas in the abdomen can obscure potential findings. Additionally, ultrasound can be painful in a setting where the patient already has abdominal pain from diverticulitis. While MRI is excellent in evaluating soft tissue, it is a much lengthier test than CT and is, therefore, unsuitable for critically ill patients, emergency cases, and patients with severe claustrophobia. It is also a poor choice for patients with instrumentation such as pacemakers and metallic implants [10].

Colonoscopy is not recommended during an acute episode of diverticulitis as it is associated with a risk of bowel perforation. However, all patients are recommended to undergo a colonoscopy postoperatively (see "Follow-Up and Postoperative Considerations" for further discussion on this topic).

## *Nonoperative Management: Antibiotics*

Uncomplicated diverticulitis is often treated on an outpatient basis with a 7–10 day course of oral broad-spectrum antibiotics, a clear liquid diet, and a follow-up in

2–3 days. Antibiotics should be chosen for the coverage of Gram-negative rods and anaerobes, the most common organisms found in the GI tract. Common antibiotics used for outpatient treatment of uncomplicated diverticulitis include trimethoprim-sulfamethoxazole or ciprofloxacin or levofloxacin with metronidazole. Table 11.1, adapted from Iida et al., provides the antibiotic regimens for treating acute diverticulitis, depending on the setting (inpatient versus outpatient) and severity of disease. Patients with more severe symptoms, such as signs of peritonitis or inability to tolerate oral intake, can be admitted to the hospital for intravenous (IV) antibiotics, IV fluid resuscitation, and bowel rest. Although antibiotics are a part of the treatment, studies have suggested that they may have limited use in acute uncomplicated diverticulitis and play a minimum role in preventing recurrence, preventing complications, or accelerating recovery [10]. Most patients experience improvement of symptoms within 48–72 h, and 50–70% have no further episodes of diverticulitis [8].

**Table 11.1** Recommended antibiotic regimens for acute diverticulitis

| Setting | Primary antibiotic regimen | Alternative regimens |
|---|---|---|
| Outpatient: mild, uncomplicated | Antibiotics not recommended | |
| Outpatient: worsening | Trimethoprim/sulfamethoxazole DS 160/800 mg PO q12 h | Amoxicillin/clavulanate ER 1000/62.5 mg, two tablets PO q12 h |
| | OR | OR |
| | Ciprofloxacin 750 mg PO q12 h or levofloxacin 750 mg PO q24 h PLUS metronidazole 500 mg PO q6 h | Moxifloxacin 400 mg PO q24 h |
| Inpatient: mild-mod | Piperacillin/tazobactam 3.375 g IV q6 h OR 4.5 g IV q8 h | Ciprofloxacin 400 mg IV q12 h or levofloxacin 750 mg IV q24 h PLUS metronidazole 500 mg IV q6 h or 1 g IV q12 h |
| | OR | OR |
| | Ticarcillin/clavulanate 3.1 g IV q6 h | Tigecycline 100 mg IV first dose, then 50 mg IV q12 h |
| | OR | OR |
| | Ertapenem 1 g IV q24 h | Moxifloxacin 400 mg IV 1 24 h |
| | OR | |
| | Moxifloxacin 400 mg IV q24 h | |
| Inpatient: severe | Imipenem/cilastatin 500 mg IV q6 h | Ampicillin 2 g IV q6 h PLUS metronidazole 500 mg IV q6 h PLUS ciprofloxacin 400 mg IV q12 h or levofloxacin 750 mg IV q24 h |
| | OR | OR |
| | Meropenem 1 g IV q8 h | Ampicillin 2 g IV q6 h PLUS metronidazole 500 mg IV q6 h PLUS amikacin, gentamicin, or tobramycin |
| | OR | |
| | Doripenem 500 mg IV q8 h | |

## Nonoperative Management: Image-Guided Percutaneous Abscess Drainage

In patients who do not improve or worsen despite treatment, complications such as abscess formation should be considered; these patients should be hospitalized and further investigated with additional imaging. Patients who are more likely to fail outpatient treatment are those who were initially found to have free fluid on CT. Diverticulitis complicated by abscess requires treatment as there is a risk of perforation, particularly in patients who are immunosuppressed and those taking NSAIDs, corticosteroids, or chronic opioids [10].

While some small abscesses (<3 cm) can be treated with antibiotics, patients who do not improve with antibiotics should be considered for other interventions. Although intra-abdominal abscesses are traditionally treated with operative drainage, image-guided percutaneous abscess drainage (IGPAD) is now the treatment of choice as it is a minimally invasive procedure with a high rate of success and can often be performed on an outpatient basis. Ultrasonography and CT are the most commonly used modalities for IGPAD, with CT-guided abscess drainage successfully treating 70–90% of intra-abdominal abscesses [11].

Prior to the procedure, the patient's imaging and laboratory parameters should be thoroughly reviewed. Laboratory tests obtained include serum coagulation parameters and serum hemoglobin levels, despite the procedure having only a moderate risk of bleeding. Dr. Hearns Charles of the NYU Langone Medical Center Section of Vascular and Interventional Radiology recommends discontinuing thienopyridines, such as clopidogrel, 5 days prior to the procedure, although aspirin can be continued. Low-molecular-weight heparin should also be withheld, depending on half-life – Charles recommends holding for 2–4 half-lives prior to the procedure [11].

Since IGPAD is considered a dirty procedure, antibiotic prophylaxis is recommended by the Society of Interventional Radiology. Although there is no consensus on a first-line antibiotic, broad-spectrum antibiotics are recommended as abscesses are generally polymicrobial. The antibiotic chosen should cover skin flora (Gram-positive bacteria) and typical intra-abscess organisms (Gram negatives). It should be administered intravenously at least 1 h prior to the procedure, and the regimen should be continued after the procedure [11].

The imaging modality selected for guidance is dependent on numerous factors. Conventional fluoroscopy by itself is a poor choice as it does not provide enough detail, so it is largely limited to drainage of large superficial abscesses. It is, however, often used as an adjunct to ultrasound- or CT-guided drainage. After successfully obtaining needle access using ultrasound or CT, serial dilatation and accurate catheter placement are often achieved through fluoroscopy guidance. Ultrasonography and fluoroscopy drainage is, in general, considered the most dynamic method as it allows for real-time visualization of needle advancement in multiple planes as well as direct visualization of placement of the dilator and catheter. Ultrasonography, however, is limited by intra-abscess air that can obscure visualization of the abscess. In these cases, CT is a superior method [11].

There are two techniques of IGPAD that can be employed, depending on the location and size of the abscess – the trocar technique and the Seldinger technique. The trocar technique is usually used for large and superficial collections and the Seldinger technique for high-risk, small, deep, and difficult to access abscesses.

**Trocar Technique** A small gauge needle is initially inserted, and the contents of the abscess are aspirated to verify correct needle placement. A catheter, stiffening cannula, and sharp stylet, in a coaxial combination, are then advanced into the collection, parallel to the initial needle.

**Seldinger Technique** A 21- or 22-gauge needle is used for initial access into the abscess cavity. A 0.018-in wire conversion to 0.035- or 0.038-in wire is then used with a Cope, Neff, or AccuStick coaxial catheter introduction system.

Although the trocar technique is correlated with more patient pain, it is faster and is associated with less abscess leakage than that associated with the serial access tract dilatation used in the Seldinger technique [11].

Regardless of the imaging modality or technique used, for accurate needle and catheter placement, it is critical to measure the distance from skin to the entry point of the abscess cavity for the initial length of the needle access. Operator feeling is also critical in detecting ease of wire, dilator, and catheter advancement. Each device should travel freely into the abscess without resistance and concurrent significant patient pain. The wire should advance into the abscess and assume the shape of the cavity. Once needle access is placed into the abscess, a specimen should be collected before injecting any contrast material. However, one should avoid aspirating the entirety of the contents before advancement of the drainage catheter, as collapse of the cavity can prevent proper catheter placement [11].

The viscosity of the abscess contents, in rare cases, can prevent successful aspiration. In these cases, a wire test can be employed to determine if the contents are drainable. If the guidewire is able to pass into the cavity, the cavity is considered, at least partially; fluid and successful aspiration should be achievable through the introduction of a dilator or drainage catheter. If the abscess contents are deemed to be undrainable, tissue plasminogen activator (tPA) can be used to facilitate drainage [11].

Potential complications of IGPAD include bleeding, hematoma, peritonitis, pseudoaneurysm formation, and sepsis. To minimize the risk of complications associated with IGPAD, Dr. Charles recommends the following:

1. Use the safest, most direct, and shortest percutaneous route.
2. Avoid intervening organs or vital anatomical structures.
3. Avoid contamination of sterile areas.
4. Aim for placing the drainage catheter in the most dependent portion of the cavity.
5. Use an angled approach. [11]

## Other Complications and Nonoperative Management

In addition to abscess formation, LBO is another complication of acute diverticulitis, occurring in 67% of patients. Complete obstruction develops in 10% of patients. Patients with incomplete obstruction are treated with and respond to fluid resuscitation and nasogastric suction. Gastrografin enemas can be used to assess if a true LBO has occurred. Patients who do not respond to nonoperative management require surgery [8].

Fistulas develop in 5% of patients with complicated diverticulitis, with colovesical fistulas being the most common [8]. It is important to rule out other causes of fistula formation, including carcinoma of the colon and adjacent organs, such as the bladder, Crohn's disease, injury resulting from pervious radiation, and trauma [9]. CT is most useful in diagnosing a colovesical fistula and in visualizing any masses or abscesses associated with the fistula and in ruling out the other causes of fistula formation. Contrast enemas and small bowel studies can help define the fistula tract. Patients with fistulas should undergo resection of the affected segment [8].

Diverticular bleeding occurs due to the erosion of an arteriole adjacent to the diverticulum and can result in hemorrhage. Bleeding resolves spontaneously in 80% of patients, and management focuses on resuscitation and localization of the bleed. Colonoscopy can be used to identify the bleed and treat it with an injection of epinephrine or with cautery [8]. Mesenteric angiography can also be used both as a diagnostic tool as well as a therapeutic intervention. It can identify the site of bleeding, and vasopressin can be instilled through to catheter at the bleeding site. Vasopressin has been shown to successfully stop over 80% of diverticular bleeds; however, over half of these cases will re-bleed. It is, therefore, used as a temporizing measure to allow for resuscitation and subsequent colon resection. Another temporizing measure commonly used is transcatheter embolization with coils. It is effective in stopping acute bleeds but is associated with a risk of bowel ischemia and infarction [9]. In rare cases of persistent or recurring hemorrhage despite nonoperative or temporizing management, the patient may require a segmental colectomy [8].

## Operative Management

Fifteen to thirty percent of hospitalized patients ultimately require surgery during the admission, whether it is laparoscopic, open, or robotic colectomies, drainage, or washouts [10]. The decision to perform surgery depends on a number of factors, including the severity of the patient's disease, the frequency of recurrences, the degree of impairment on the patient's life, and patient factors, including comorbidities and medications [12]. Emergency surgery may be required if an abscess is unable to be drained percutaneously, if the patient's clinical status fails to improve or worsens, or if the patient has peritonitis. Studies have also shown that laparoscopic lavage and drainage without bowel resection may also be effective; however, this approach is not yet recommended for most cases as it requires additional prospective trials [8]. Emergent colectomy is known to be associated with significant morbidity, including pneumonia, respiratory failure, myocardial infection, as well as increased mortality in the elderly [10].

## Emergency Surgery

The goal of emergency treatment is to stabilize the patient. This may include conservative treatment or abscess drainage, abdominal lavage, and/or sigmoid colon resection. Emergency surgery is required for patients with multi-quadrant peritonitis, Hinchey stage III or IV disease, or bowel perforation. Patients usually appear acutely ill or toxic and should be immediately treated with fluid resuscitation, antibiotics, and operative management. Historically, Hartmann's procedure with creation of an end colostomy is the operation of choice. However, given that this procedure usually requires a second operation to reverse the stoma and anastamose the descending colon to the rectum, many are considering primary resection and anastomosis with or without stoma as an alternative. Additionally, studies have found an improved quality of life after primary anastomosis. The decision on which procedure to use depends on the patient's risk profile. In patients with multiple comorbidities, severe sepsis, or prolonged feculent peritonitis, Hartmann's procedure is preferred. Otherwise, in relatively healthy patients, it is reasonable to consider a primary anastomosis with or without a diverting proximal stoma. In many cases, a sigmoidectomy is avoided altogether, and a lavage and drainage is done instead. One study successfully treated 95.7% of patients with laparoscopic lavage and drainage alone. Laparoscopic surgery is preferred over the open approach when emergently treating for Hinchey stage III and IV acute complicated diverticulitis [13].

## Elective Sigmoidectomy

A sigmoidectomy with primary anastomosis is the elective procedure of choice for diverticulitis. It is optimally performed 6–8 weeks after an episode of acute diverticulitis, during the inflammation-free period. Studies have found that surgeries done during this period lead to better results than those done during the "early elective" period, with lower rates of anastomotic leaks, wound infections, and laparoscopic cases necessitating conversion to open surgery [12]. Surgery is generally recommended after the first episode of complicated diverticulitis, as there is a high risk of recurrent disease [13]. This is especially true for younger patients (age 50 or younger), as the risk of complications increase with each recurrence; however, recent guidelines no longer recommend earlier resection in younger patients [14].

Traditionally, an elective sigmoidectomy was also indicated after two episodes of uncomplicated diverticulitis; however, some studies suggest that surgery should be delayed until after the third or fourth episode to reduce the overall number of surgeries a patient may receive without increasing the risk of complications, such as diverticular perforation [15]. Additionally, the number of episodes may not even be associated with the risk of complications. As a result, today, the number of episodes alone does not indicate the need for surgery [12]. According to the American Society of Colon and Rectal Surgery, "the number of attacks of uncomplicated diverticulitis is not necessarily an overriding factor in defining the appropriateness of surgery" [15]. The most cost-effective approach has been found to be pursuing surgery after the third episode of acute uncomplicated diverticulitis requiring hospitalization; however, the decision should be individualized based on patient factors including patient preference, comorbidities, and lifestyle [10]. It is important to consider each individual patient's risk factors, as those with increased risk of recurrence or complications, such as patients who are immunosuppressed, may benefit more from early elective surgery [12].

There is an increased incidence of diverticulitis in immunosuppressed patients compared to the general population (1% vs. 0.02%). These patients also tend to experience much more severe disease, as immunosuppression and steroid intake are known risk factors for perforation. As a result, emergency surgery is performed in 80–90% of these patients experiencing their first episode of diverticulitis. In patients who were diagnosed with diverticulosis before the onset of immunosuppression, 16% of them developed diverticulitis while immunosuppressed. This has led to suggestions of performing elective surgery in these patients before they develop diverticulitis. Brandl et al. studied 227 patients who were treated for diverticulitis in an inpatient setting, 15 of whom were immunocompromised (on immunosuppressive medications or post-solid organ transplantation). The study found a higher rate of complicated diverticulitis and subsequent emergency surgeries, longer ICU stays, longer hospitalizations, and higher hospital mortality in immunosuppressed patients. The study was limited by the small number of subjects examined and by the retrospective design; therefore, it is difficult to draw general recommendations on treating diverticulitis in immunosuppressed patients. However, given the high rates of diverticulitis complications in immunosuppressed patients, diverticulosis itself may be an indication for elective surgery – the goal in these patients is to prevent diverticulitis before it ever occurs [16].

## Colectomy

Surgical treatment of diverticulitis is often curative and has a recurrence rate of less than 5% [15]. The principle of surgery for treating diverticulitis is complete removal of all the inflamed or affected segments of the bowel, most commonly the sigmoid colon. The resection should distally extend to the rectum, even if the sigmoid is not affected, as there is a high rate of recurrence if part of the sigmoid is retained.

Removing all diverticula in the remaining colon, however, is not necessary since the number of diverticula does not correlate with risk of recurrence or progression [12]. Nevertheless, it is important to avoid including any diverticula into the stapled colorectal anastomosis. The anastomosis should be made between the descending colon and the upper rectum. Some surgeons prefer to preserve the inferior mesenteric artery as it may minimize the risk of anastomotic leak and sexual dysfunction secondary to nerve injury [15]. The surgery can be done open or minimally invasively.

Laparoscopic surgery has largely replaced the open approach for the elective treatment of diverticulitis. Compared to the open approach, laparoscopic sigmoidectomy is associated with shorter hospitalization, more rapid return of bowel function, decreased morbidity, and lower costs [12]. It is also associated with less blood loss [17]. Additionally, there is significant reduction in major complications, including intra-abdominal abscesses, anastomotic leaks, pulmonary embolism, and myocardial infarction [15]. Laparoscopic surgery has been found to have lower mortality during hospitalization compared to open surgery [10]. Laparoscopic sigmoidectomies are performed using 4–5 ports, depending on whether there is need to mobilize the splenic flexure. Through these ports, the sigmoid colon is dissected medially to laterally, and the mesentery up to the descending colon is mobilized [17]. The bowel is then resected using a surgical stapler, and the specimen is delivered through one of the port incisions. A primary colorectal anastomosis is usually performed; however, some patients may require the creation of an end colostomy.

Another minimally invasive approach is a robotic colectomy. Bhama et al. conducted a study in 2016 to compare the outcomes of colorectal procedures done laparoscopically versus robotically. Compared to the laparoscopic approach, the robotic method was found to have lower rates of conversion to open procedures for pelvic cases (up to 10% versus up to 34% in laparoscopic cases). Some analyses have also shown decreased length of hospital stay in patients who undergo robotic procedures, both abdominal and pelvic. Although operative times were longer for robotic procedures, there were no differences in postoperative complications observed between the two groups of patients. Additionally, operative times were found to depend on surgeon experience and improve with increased experience [18]. A study by D'Annibale et al. also found no difference in actual operative time between their laparoscopic and robotic groups; rather the robotic cases had longer preparation times [19].

Robotic cases are most commonly performed with multiple incisions, allowing for flexibility and space for the maneuver of instruments; however, they can be done with a single incision as well. In patients who are appropriate candidates, single-incision colectomy allows for effective resection of the bowel with improved cosmesis compared to multiple incision cases. Ideal candidates for single-incision robotic colectomies are patients with a body mass index (BMI) less than 25 and, in cases of colonic tumors, patients with small tumors (stages T1–3). Patients with higher BMIs are at increased risk of complications postoperatively [20].

With colectomies, one must decide between a primary anastomosis and performing a Hartmann procedure with the creation of an end colostomy. Although a primary anastomosis is typically the procedure of choice, the decision is dependent on the patient's severity of disease. For Hinchey stages I and II, where the patient has only small localized abscesses, a primary anastomosis is usually performed. For larger abscesses or patients with peritonitis, a colectomy with end colostomy and Hartmann's pouch would be more appropriate. In these patients, a Hartmann take-down with colostomy closure and secondary colorectal anastomosis may be pursued later [8]. This typically occurs around 3 months after the initial surgery [9].

## Complications

In a systematic review and meta-analysis by Haas et al., the overall postoperative mortality rate for diverticulitis is 3.05%. In patients who underwent emergent surgery, the mortality was 10.64%, while patients who received elective surgery had a mortality of 0.5%. Laparoscopy was also associated with a lower mortality at 0.75% compared to the 4.69% rate of the open approach. In patients who received a primary anastomosis, the mortality was 1.96%. The Hartmann's procedure with an end colostomy was found to have a mortality of 14.18%. Patients who had more severe disease also experienced higher mortality – those with Hinchey classes I and II were found to have a mortality of 2.05% compared to 7.87% in those with Hinchey classes III and IV. Overall, there is a 32.64% postoperative complication rate. Postoperative complications include intra-abdominal abscesses (3.59%), bleeding (2.13%), anastomotic leak (3.99%), wound infection (6.78%), wound dehiscence (2.16%), pneumonia (3.7%), urinary tract infections (3.12%), pulmonary embolism (0.83%), and myocardial infarction (1.4%). Patients who underwent emergency surgery experienced a greater rate of complications at 53.6% than those who received elective surgery (22.52%), and patients who received laparoscopic surgery saw fewer complications than those who underwent open surgery (22.48% vs. 41.26%). Additionally, resection with a primary anastomosis resulted in a 27.62% complication rate as opposed to 40.55% seen with the Hartmann's procedure [21].

In patients who undergo robotic surgery, there are unique complications that are not seen in open or laparoscopic cases. A problem commonly discussed is the lack of tactile sensation available to the surgeon in robotic cases and the possibility of causing organ injury. However, this problem can be mitigated by careful observation of the instruments during the operation as well as the improvements that have been made in robotic technology, allowing for three-dimensional views and "visual haptic sense" that permits the surgeon to visualize how much pressure is being applied to the tissue [19].

## Follow-Up and Postoperative Considerations

Given that locally perforated colon carcinoma presents similarly to diverticulitis, all patients should undergo a colonoscopy 6 weeks after recovery, regardless if they were treated nonoperatively or if they underwent surgery [10].

Diverticulitis has a recurrence rate of 9–36% in patients treated nonoperatively, with patients aged 50 and older experiencing lower risk of recurrence than younger patients. To prevent recurrence, there are many lifestyle changes that patients can make, including increased fiber intake and/or use of fiber supplements, regular physical activity, weight loss, and smoking cessation. Some studies have also demonstrated that mesalamine, *Lactobacillus casei*, and rifaximin, in addition to fiber, can help prevent recurrence, contribute to symptom relief, and lower the risk of complications [10].

# References

1. Gingold D, Murrell Z. Management of colonic volvulus. Clin Colon Rectal Surg. 2012;25(4):236–44.
2. Bhimji SS, Cooper W. Volvulus. StatPearls [Internet]. Treasure Island (FL): StatPearls Publishing. 2017. Retrieved from https://www.ncbi.nlm.nih.gov/books/NBK441836/
3. Lieske B, Antunes C. Sigmoid Volvulus. StatPearls [Internet]. Treasure Island (FL): StatPearls Publishing. 2017. Retrieved from https://www.ncbi.nlm.nih.gov/books/NBK441925/
4. Akinkuotu A, Samuel JC, Msiska N, Mvula C, Charles AG. The role of the anatomy of the sigmoid Colon in developing sigmoid volvulus: a case-control study. Clin Anat. 2011;24(5):634–7. https://doi.org/10.1002/ca.21131.
5. Ballantyne GH, Brandner MD, Beart RW, Ilstrup DM. Volvulus of the Colon: incidence and mortality. Ann Surg. 1985;202(1):83–92.
6. Scharl M, Biedermann L. A symptomatic coffee bean: acute sigmoid volvulus. Case Rep Gastroenterol. 2017;11(2):348–51.
7. Iida T, Nakagaki S, Satoh S, Shimizu H, Kaneto H, Nakase H. Clinical outcomes of sigmoid colon volvulus: identification of the factors associated with successful endoscopic detorsion. Intest Res. 2017;15(2):215–20. https://doi.org/10.5217/ir.2017.15.2.215.
8. Bullard Dunn KM, Rothenberger DA. Colon, rectum, and anus. In: Brunicardi F, Andersen DK, Billiar TR, Dunn DL, Hunter JG, Matthews JB, Pollock RE, editors. Schwartz's principles of surgery, 10e. New York: McGraw-Hill; 2015. p. 1189–203.
9. Dayton MT, Isenberg GA, Rakinic J, et al. Colon, rectum, and anus. In: Lawrence PF, editor. Essentials of general surgery, 5e. Baltimore: Lippincott Williams & Wilkins; 2013. p. 307–9.
10. Wilkins T, Embry K, George R. Diagnosis and management of acute diverticulitis. Am Fam Physician. 2013;87(9):612–20.
11. Charles HW. Abscess drainage. Semin Intervent Radiol. 2012;29:325–36.
12. Jurowich CF, Germer CT. Elective surgery for sigmoid diverticulitis – indications, techniques, and results. Viszeralmedizin. 2015;31:112–6.
13. Kockerling F. Emergency surgery for acute complicated diverticulitis. Viszeralmedizin. 2015;31:107–10.
14. Simianu VV, Fichera A, Bastawrous AL, Davidson GH, Florence MG, Thirlby RC, et al. Number of diverticulitis episodes before resection and factors associated with earlier interventions. JAMA Surg. 2016;151(7):604–10.
15. Stocchi L. Current indications and role of surgery in the management of sigmoid diverticulitis. World J Gastroenterol. 2010;16(7):804–17.
16. Brandl A, Kratzer T, Kafka-Ritsch R, Braunwarth E, Denecke C, Weiss S, et al. Diverticulitis in immunosuppressed patients: a fatal outcome requiring a new approach? Can J Surg. 2016;59(4):254–61.
17. Siddiqui MRS, Sajid MS, Khatri K, Cheek E, Baig MK. Elective open versus laparoscopic sigmoid colectomy for diverticular disease: a meta-analysis with the sigma trial. World J Surg. 2010;34:2883–901.

18. Bhama AR, Obias V, Welch KB, Vandewarker JF, Cleary RK. A comparison of laparoscopic and robotic colorectal surgery outcomes using the American College of Surgeons National Surgical Quality Improvement Program (ACS NSQIP) database. Surg Endosc. 2015;30:1576–84. https://doi.org/10.1007/s00464-015-4381-9.
19. Ramamoorthy S, Obias V. Unique complications of robotic colorectal surgery. Surg Clin North Am. 2013;93:273–86. https://doi.org/10.1016/j.suc.2012.09.01.
20. Skancke M, Obias V. Single incision robotic colorectal surgery: history, indications, and techniques for success with single incision colectomy. Seminars in Colon and Rectal Surgery. 2016;27:166–9. https://doi.org/10.1053/j.scrs.2016.04.010.
21. Haas JM, Singh M, Vakil N. Mortality and complications following surgery for diverticulitis: systematic review and meta-analysis. United European Gastroenterol J. 2015;4(5):703–13.

# Chapter 12
# Minimally Invasive Hernia Surgery

Karl A. LeBlanc and Zinda Z. LeBlanc

## Introduction

Minimally invasive surgery (MIS) methods have been used in operative procedures for many decades. Until the late 1980s, there had been little adoption into the general surgery operations but wide adoption in the gynecologic procedures. While a few general surgeons used laparoscopy for diagnostic procedures and liver biopsy, there were little perceived opportunities in this area. The performance of the first laparoscopic cholecystectomy in 1987 changed the mindset of the surgical world. This led to a rapid adoption of this minimally invasive tool and a rapid response from industry to facilitate the instrumentation necessary to advance these methods.

Minimally invasive hernia surgery was a logical operation to the average general surgeon. The first inguinal hernia was actually performed by Dr. Fletcher as early as 1976, but the first report was by Ralph Ger in 1982 [1]. The first laparoscopic incisional hernia repair was performed in 1991 and reported in 1993 by this author [2]. Currently these procedures are now performed routinely across the globe, but its usage varies significantly from country to country. The number of inguinal repairs performed is 10–60% in developed countries. In contrast, the incisional hernia repair rate is 5–35%. An even smaller number of robot-assisted repairs of each of these problems are presently done. The USA leads in the number of surgeons that utilize the robot for hernia repair.

K. A. LeBlanc (✉)
Department of Surgery, Our Lady of the Lake Regional Medical Center, Baton Rouge, LA, USA

Z. Z. LeBlanc
Woman's Hospital of Baton Rouge, Baton Rouge, LA, USA
e-mail: zinda.leblanc@womans.org

© Springer Nature Switzerland AG 2019                                                  155
C. Rezac, K. Donohue (eds.), *The Internist's Guide to Minimally Invasive Gastrointestinal Surgery*, Clinical Gastroenterology,
https://doi.org/10.1007/978-3-319-96631-1_12

The selection of a minimally invasive approach will be determined by the ability of the general surgeon to perform the procedure. Frequently (and not unexpectedly) if that surgeon does not have the skill set to perform them, then this will not be offered as an option to the patient. It must not be overlooked, however, that there are concerns that will be patient and/or facility specific. Many patients are not candidates for minimally invasive techniques, or the facility does not support the technical requirements of these procedures. Consequently, the use of MIS hernia repair will be determined by a multitude of factors.

This chapter will develop the advantages and disadvantages of these MIS options. Patient selection and preoperative and postoperative expectations will be discussed with particular attention to the knowledge beneficial to the treating internal medicine physician. The reader is referred to the numerous hardcopy or online materials and videos that are available if further information is desired.

## Preoperative Issues

Generally speaking, if the patient can undergo a general anesthetic, he or she can be considered for a MIS hernia repair. While the inguinal hernia repair has been performed under epidural anesthesia, this is very seldom considered as an option as these patients must be placed in a steep Trendelenburg position, which can compromise the respiratory status of the patient, and necessary relaxation during surgery may not be reliably achieved. Very large inguinal hernias are particularly difficult in the MIS method as the reduction of hernia contents may be problematic or impossible due to long-standing adhesions of bowel to the hernia sac itself. In many cases, the use of MIS in the obese or morbidly obese patient is preferred due to the lower risk of the development of venous thrombosis and a significantly lower incidence of wound infection. There are opinions that patients with high BMI should lose weight to achieve a BMI < 50 prior to surgery to decrease risk and improve outcomes most especially for ventral and incisional hernias [3]. In all cases, it is recommended if the patient stops smoking at least 4 weeks prior to the operation to minimize the chronic cough of smokers, to decrease the risk of wound infection, and to allow for proper healing to occur.

The preoperative workup of an inguinal hernia patient will be minimal for the individual with few medical problems. Usually a complete blood count, comprehensive metabolic panel, and an electrocardiogram (if over 50 years old) will suffice. For those higher-risk patients, any metabolic derangements should be controlled to the best extent possible. Anticoagulants must be stopped in enough time to negate their effects. Despite appropriate cessation of these agents, these patients are still at higher risk of postoperative bleeding, which will sometimes make the MIS choice a less attractive option. If the patient cannot stop these agents (e.g., a fresh cardiac artery stent), the MIS repair has a very high risk of significant postoperative hemorrhage. Most surgeons will opt for an open repair in these situations.

Most small- to medium-sized ventral and incisional hernias can be repaired with the MIS method. The size would vary according to other issues such as the comorbidities of the patient. While some hernias may externally appear to be massive, the actual fascial defect to be repaired may be much smaller. Although the actual dimensions that can be approached this way will vary from surgeon to surgeon, a rough estimate of fascial defect size will be less than 6–8 cm in transverse dimension. A "gray area" of size is from 6 to 10 cm, but nearly all defects larger than 10 cm will be approached by an open method rather than a MIS technique.

Considerations of the MIS repair for ventral and incisional hernias differ from those of the inguinal hernias. These patients are often at higher risk due to more frequent presence of common ailments that need to be addressed or corrected preoperatively. In particular, smoking cessation of 1 month is often felt to be so important as to delay elective surgery if the patient does not stop. This is often verified by either blood or breathe tests. The patients with these types of hernia need good venous return and should not have significant heart failure during the procedure. The required abdominal insufflation may delay venous return and affect cardiac function. Preoperative cardiac evaluation is often required in patients suspected of such an issue.

Diabetes mellitus must be controlled. Ideally, the hemoglobin A1c should be no more than eight, but closer to normal is preferred. Tissue healing is impaired if these levels are higher than the accepted range. On the day of surgery, it is accepted practice to check the glucose level in the preoperative holding area. If this level is exceedingly high such as 300 or more, the surgery will often be cancelled or at least delayed until this can be treated. A concern of an untreated infection that is signaled by this high glucose level can also dictate further therapy.

Of course, optimization of all medical conditions is preferred for all surgical procedures that are considered elective. Patients with significant lung disease may not be candidates for MIS surgery, but often these patients fare better with these approaches rather than the open surgical option. If there is significant right heart failure, the use of the intra-abdominal insufflation pressures could adversely affect venous return. Unless the patient has an active exacerbation of problems such as sarcoidosis or lupus, control of these processes will allow the procedure to proceed.

The use of corticosteroids before and after these operations is not considered ideal. If these cannot be stopped, then preoperative boost doses of these drugs will be administered on the day of surgery and afterwards as deemed necessary. Steroids impede healing. All MIS hernia repairs rely on the use of a prosthetic mesh of some type. Tissue ingrowth into these materials will vary depending upon the product selected. Patients not on steroids will have enough tissue penetration in these products by 6 weeks in most cases as to allow normal activities. The surgeon will have to determine if this postoperative time should be extended to 90 days or more based upon such factors such as hernia type, mesh size, mesh type, or method of mesh fixation.

## Prosthetic Implants Used in Hernioplasty

This chapter is not meant to be an exhaustive compilation of the numerous materials that are available for the repair of hernias. The purpose of a mesh is to support the weakened tissue that has allowed the development of a defect in the fascia. The addition of a mesh rather than suture alone lowers the recurrence rates of incisional hernia by half [4, 5]. It would seem that a very basic understanding of the uses and other considerations of these materials that are used in the repair of MIS hernias should be known by nonsurgeons. In most cases, the meshes that can be used in the laparoscopic methods can also be used in the open methods. However, many products have been developed that are specifically designed for use in the MIS technique. This is especially true for inguinal hernia repair. A broad segregation of these products can be into absorbable, nonabsorbable, synthetic, or non-synthetic materials. If more information is desired, the reader is referred to the actual manufacturer, the Internet, or recently published material [6]. The products discussed below are examples of such materials, and their inclusion in this chapter serves as examples of such products and represents neither an exhaustive list nor an endorsement of the product.

Absorbable synthetic products are used in circumstances where the implantation of a permanent material is ill advised. Such situations occur when an active infection exists at the area of the hernia itself. Alternatively, these can be used as a temporary repair in such cases where the patient may require multiple returns to the operating room such as in trauma. Older products are Vicryl (Ethicon, Inc., Somerville, NJ, USA) and Dexon (Medtronic, Minneapolis, MN, USA) meshes. The more recent materials that are most often used in the USA are Bio-A (W. L. Gore & Associates, Elkhart, DE) and Phasix (CR Bard, Providence, RI, USA). There is some evidence that the former product can result in a permanent repair [7]. Ongoing research indicates that these materials may be appropriate for the permanent repair of fascial defects, but more studies are needed to verify this claim.

Biologic products are also not a permanent material but differ in the absorbable meshes in that all of them are produced from a once-living organism. These are obtained from bovine, porcine, or cadaveric sources. Generally the dermis of the animal is harvested and processed to produce a flat sheet of white material to be used in the repair of tissue defects. Other sources of tissue are the small intestine or stomach. The concept is that these meshes will act as a scaffold for collagen deposition and will ultimately be replaced by native collagen of the patient. Although these are most often placed during open surgery, they are sometimes used in laparoscopic applications. Strattice RTM (Acelity, San Antonio, TX, USA) is a porcine dermal product that is commonly used. XenMatrix AB (Davol, Inc., Warwick, RI, USA) is a unique porcine dermal product that contains minocycline and rifampin as antimicrobial agents. The rifampin imparts an orange color (Fig. 12.1).

Recent product developments have resulted in the production of products that are a combination of synthetic absorbable and permanent materials. The materials currently available are OviTex (TELA Bio, Malvern, PA, USA), Synecor (W. L. Gore

**Fig. 12.1** XenMatrix AB

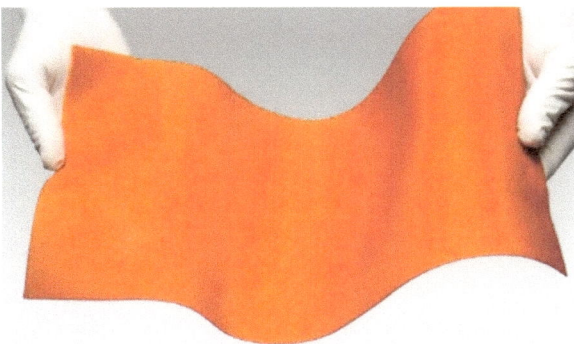

**Fig. 12.2** Synecor

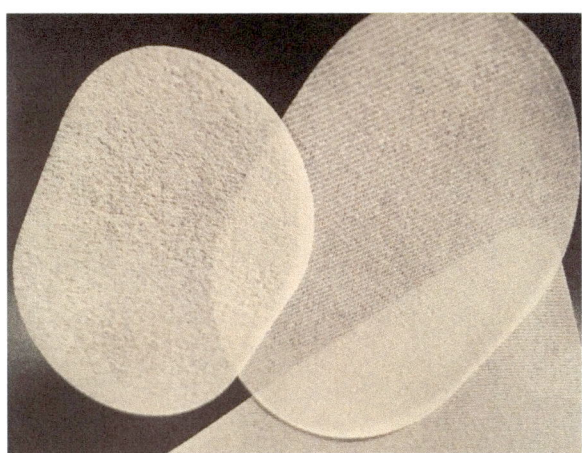

& Associates, Elkhart, DE, USA), and Zenapro (Cook Medical, Bloomington, IL, USA). The absorbable portion acts as a scaffold to increase collagen deposition. The permanent material lies between the layers of the absorbable product and remains to act as the traditional mesh repair (Fig. 12.2). OviTex and Zenapro use ovine gastric submucosa and porcine small intestinal submucosa, respectively, while the Synecor uses Bio-A/polyglycolic acid/trimethylene carbonate as the non-permanent material.

There is a large selection of permanent sheets of mesh that can be used in the repair of hernias. In general, a "nonprotected" mesh is used for inguinal hernia repair. This "nonprotected" term refers to the fact that there is no coating on the product to prevent ingrowth of tissue. A "protected" mesh is one that is coated on one side to restrict or separate tissue penetration. These are most commonly used in the repair of ventral and incisional hernias when the mesh is placed in the intraperitoneal position. The base structure of all of these products is polypropylene, polyester, or polytetra-fluoroethylene. These can be manufactured into several different weaves, shapes, or types. The coatings on the protected meshes are made of a multitude of different

**Fig. 12.3** Ventralight ST

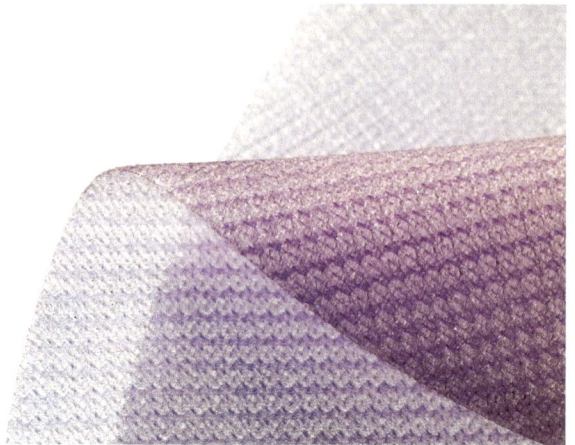

**Fig. 12.4** Symbotex

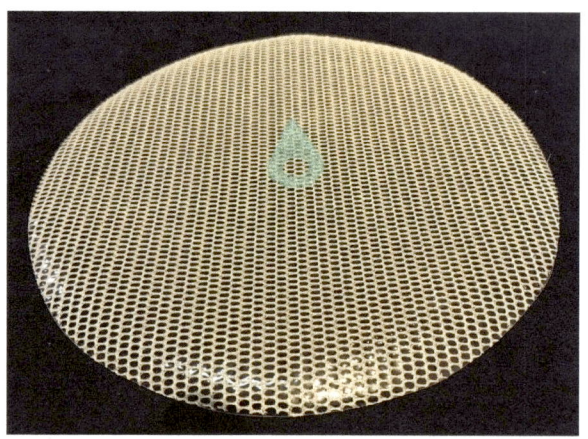

products that will absorb within 2–4 weeks in most cases (Figs. 12.3 and 12.4). Examples of these "protected" materials are Ventralight ST (Davol, Inc., Warwick, RI, USA) and Symbotex (Medtronic, Minneapolis, MN, USA). Other products are manufactured with coatings that do not absorb at all and remain on the base product or are part of the base product (Figs. 12.5 and 12.6). Examples of these are DualMesh PLUS (W. L. Gore &Associates, Elkhart, DE, USA) and DynaMesh IPOM (FEG Textiltechnik mbH, Aachen, Germany). The former product has the antimicrobial agent silver (which imparts the brown color) and chlorhexidine.

The MIS repair of inguinal repair has resulted in the development of products of many different shapes, sizes, and types. Recurrences can occur if the product is sized too small, so most of these are approximately 10 cm × 15 cm. The 3D Max (Davol, Inc., Warwick, RI, USA) has a shape designed to conform to the convexity of the inguinal floor (Fig. 12.7). The letter "M" and the arrow are placed to denote the medial placement of the mesh. The Lap ProGrip Anatomic (Medtronic,

**Fig. 12.5** DualMesh PLUS

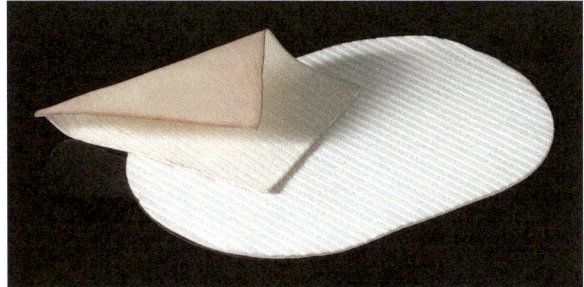

**Fig. 12.6** DynaMesh IPOM

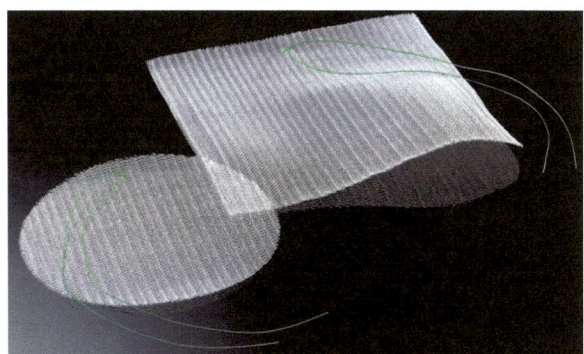

**Fig. 12.7** 3D Max

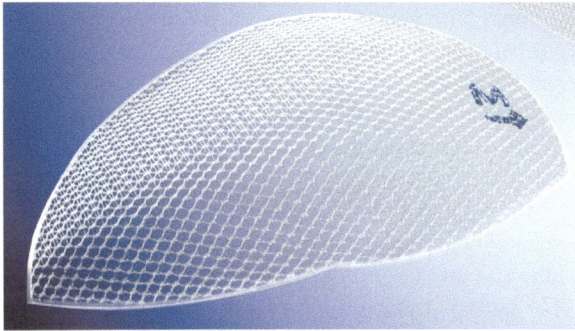

Minneapolis, MN, USA) mesh has an apron to cover the posterior aspect of the inguinal floor (Fig. 12.8). Additionally, it has "microgrips" that function like Velcro to obviate the need for suture fixation of the material.

## Inguinal Hernia Surgery

Patient selection, as with all surgical procedures, should be individualized as noted above. If the patient has had multiple prior abdominal surgeries, the MIS approach

**Fig. 12.8** Lap ProGrip
Anatomic

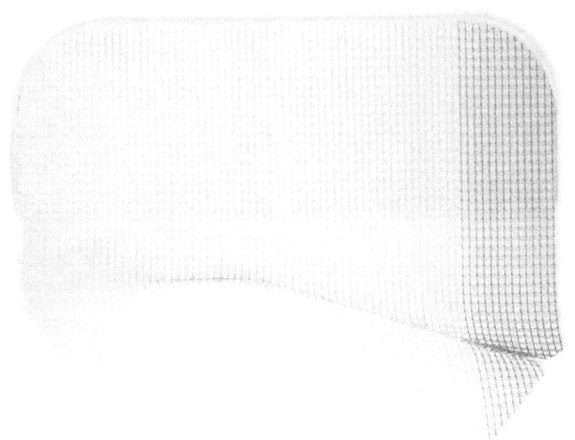

can be difficult or contraindicated if there are multiple and dense adhesions. The surgeon could elect to perform a diagnostic laparoscopic examination of the patient prior to making the final decision to proceed with the laparoscopic approach. Prior prostatectomy or laparoscopic inguinal hernia repair are relative contraindications, but this can still be performed in many cases. The incidence of chronic postoperative pain is lower with the MIS approach compared to the open techniques [8].

It is considered best if there is a discussion of the possibility of a future prostatectomy with patients that are at risk of the development of this problem. Although a prostatectomy can still be performed after laparoscopic inguinal hernia repair, it can be challenging to the urologist if they are not familiar with the postoperative anatomy. Other pelvic surgery (e.g., vascular surgery) can also be affected but not nearly as much as the prostatectomy. This does not contraindicate the procedure, however.

In this operation, the patient is placed supine on the operating table and given general endotracheal anesthesia in most cases [1, 9, 10]. The use of a nasogastric tube and urinary drainage catheter will be based upon the decision of the surgeon. The latter is frequently used if the procedure is to be more difficult than the usual case. After this has been done, the trocars will be introduced and the operative field inspected. The patient will be placed in the Trendelenburg position at that point.

There are basically two different approaches to the MIS repair. The older procedure is the transabdominal preperitoneal approach (TAPP). This requires the entry into the abdominal cavity by the operating trocars. The other approach is the totally extraperitoneal (TEP). In this method, the abdominal cavity is not entered, but the dissection of the extraperitoneal tissue is the same for both methods. The other significant difference between these approaches is that the peritoneum must be cut away from the abdominal wall in the TAPP but is not in the TEP. In both, three trocars are used. These will be placed either across the abdomen transversely or in the midline (Fig. 12.9). As noted in the diaphragm, the robotic locations are above the

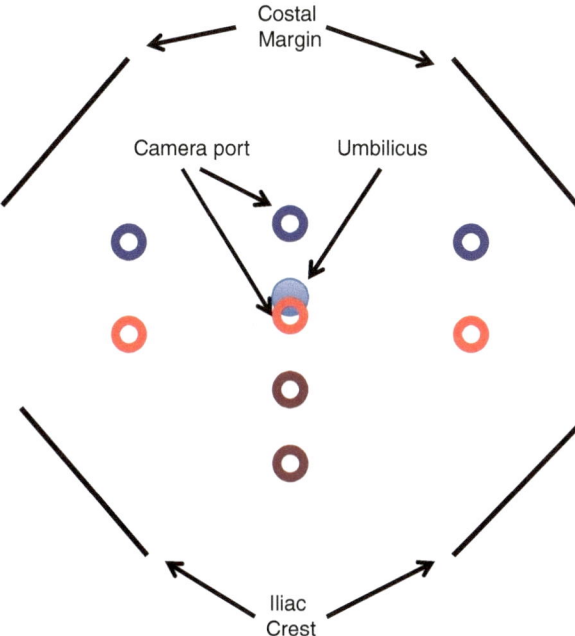

**Fig. 12.9** Typical trocar locations for laparoscopic inguinal hernia repair. Red and brown circles indicate laparoscopic locations. Blue circles indicate robot-assisted laparoscopic locations

umbilicus compared to the level of the umbilicus for the laparoscopic approach. This is required due to the fact that the robotic arms need to be further from the operative area. Additionally, the robotic approach is the TAPP and not the TEP currently.

After gaining access to the operative area, the steps of the operation are identical. The preperitoneal tissue must be separated to expose the inguinal floor. This can be challenging for some surgeons, as the anatomy is quite different than the open approach. The goal is the exposure of the entire myopectineal orifice. This orifice is the anatomic area through which all inguinal and femoral hernias occur. It is bounded by Cooper's ligament (periosteum of the pubic bone) and rectus sheath medially, the psoas muscle laterally, and the fibers of the internal oblique and transversus abdominis anteriorly. The iliopubic tract crosses this orifice (Fig. 12.10).

If this is a unilateral hernia, the dissection will be limited to the one side but will extend to both sides if bilateral. The exposure of the area is considered complete if the midline is crossed at the symphysis pubis and the dissection allows placement of the selected mesh material (Fig. 12.11). The prosthetic will be placed onto this area and sewn or tacked into place. The suture and tacks that are selected can be either permanent or absorbable. The common tack is "corkscrew"-like and is made of titanium and visible on radiographs (Fig. 12.12). These are shown as the two on the right of the photo. These as well as the FasTouch (Via Surgical, Tel Aviv, Israel) on the left are permanent products. The other devices in the photo are absorbable. There are many other types of devices available for fixation of mesh that are not shown in the figure. The use of fixation devices (which is required) has been noted to result in an increased incidence of chronic postoperative pain [11, 12].

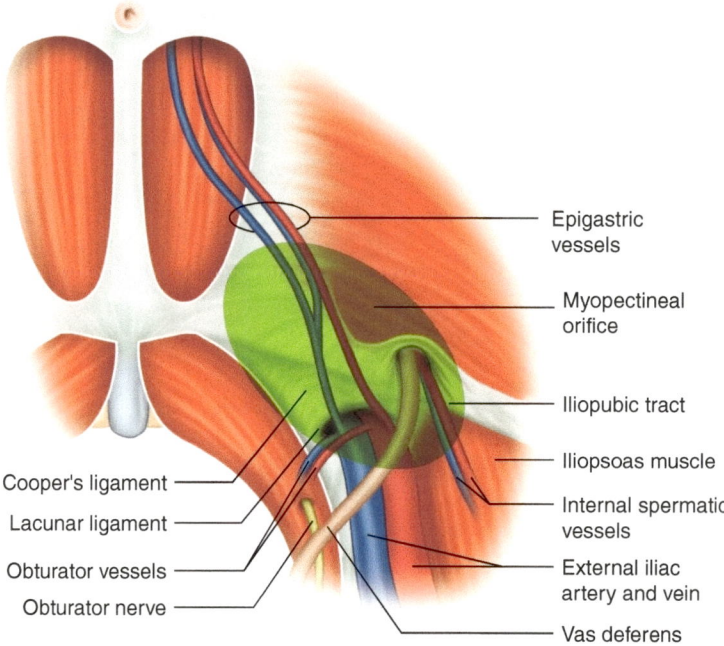

**Fig. 12.10** Myopectineal orifice

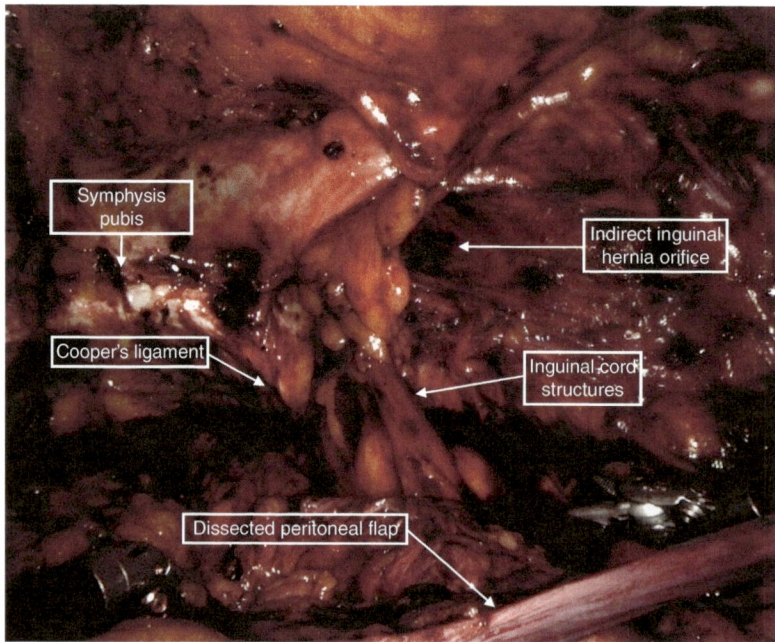

**Fig. 12.11** Dissected inguinal floor

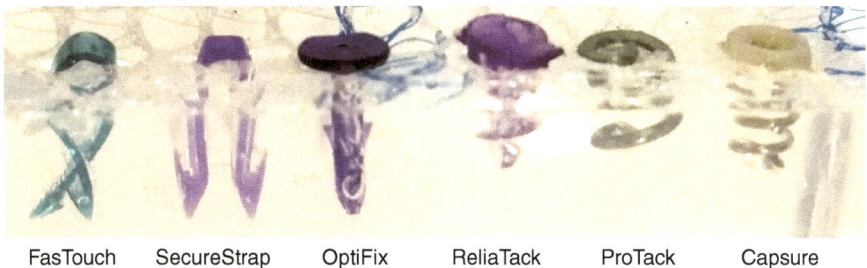

FasTouch      SecureStrap      OptiFix      ReliaTack      ProTack      Capsure

**Fig. 12.12**  Track comparison

If the TEP method has been chosen, there is no need for closure of the perito-neum, as this has not been violated. The trocars will be removed and the tissues sutured together. If the TAPP has been chosen, after mesh fixation, the peritoneum must be closed. This can be sutured or closed with one of the fixation devices. After this has been done, the trocars are removed and tissues closed. These procedures are considered outpatient surgery, so the patient will be recovered in the postanesthesia unit and then sent home.

During all laparoscopic procedures, the abdomen is insufflated with carbon diox-ide to provide working room within the abdominal cavity to perform the intended procedure. The patient will absorb this within the first 24 h in nearly all cases. If there is residual $CO_2$ within the abdomen, it will elevate under the right diaphragm resulting in referred pain in the right shoulder. This will resolve quickly but until this occurs, the patient can experience significant pain. Assumption of the supine position will cause the $CO_2$ to move to the anterior abdominal wall and relieve the shoulder pain.

Most herniologists allow the patient to perform all duties and activities of daily living as the postoperative pain allows. In general, the patient will experience only a few days of pain. It will be at the trocar sites and usually above the area of the hernia. As noted below, the use of fixation devices will influence the degree and length of time this is experienced. Extreme labor requirements and/or patient safety will influence the exact recommendation by the surgeon.

The patient will experience the persistence of a bulge or firm area at the site of the hernia that is repaired. This will occur because the tissues have been distended by the hernia itself and will occasionally result in the development of a postopera-tive seroma. This will resolve in a few weeks to a few months depending on the size and long-standing nature of the hernia preoperatively. The patient needs reassurance that this is a normal phenomenon. Even more extreme and disconcerting to the patient is the frequent occurrence of severe ecchymosis. This usually is the result of the fact that the expected hemorrhage during the operation is not removed from the patient. This blood will gravitate to the dependent portions of the patient's anatomy. This can result in large areas of bruising including the penis and scrotum. These patients must also be reassured that this is not an unexpected outcome and will resolve just like any other site of ecchymosis.

As noted earlier, one of the most common long-term complications related to inguinal hernia repair is that of chronic pain. In fact, this is more common than the

**Table 12.1** Predictors of chronic groin pain

| |
| --- |
| Young age |
| Female gender |
| Direct hernia |
| Lichtenstein or plug (open) repair |
| Bilateral repair |
| Postoperative complications |

rate of recurrence. Predictors of chronic pain postoperatively are shown in Table 12.1 [13]. As noted, the open repair is a risk factor. What is also known is that if the patient has pain preoperatively, there is a 16X greater chance that there will be chronic pain postoperatively than if no preoperative pain existed. There is no apparent difference in the occurrence of chronic pain between the TAPP and TEP unless there are more than ten tacks used [14]. If >10 are used, there is a statistically significant increase of chronic pain. In that paper, there was no difference in recurrence rates between the approaches (TEP 0.42% vs. TAPP 1.34%).

The patient with this problem should be referred to the operating surgeon. Occasionally referral to pain management will be required, but many other options exist to treat these problems. Nonsteroidal agents, gabapentin, physical therapy, and dry needling can all be used to treat this problem. If this all fails, the patient should be referred to a surgeon familiar with this problem if the operating surgeon has exhausted his or her options. The last option will be excision of the mesh and fixation devices, but even this does not resolve the pain in all cases [15]. Included in that operation will be a neurectomy of the three involved nerves. These nerves are sensory only and no motor functions will be affected. Few patients will even experience permanent numbness due to the multiple courses and interconnections of the nerves in this area.

Despite the best efforts of the surgeon, failure of the repair does occur. There are many technical factors that can predispose to recurrence. In general, if such a problem occurs, this will become evident within 1 year of the surgery. These factors include poor dissection of the operative area, improper sizing of the mesh, inadequate fixation, curling of the mesh, etc. These issues will seldom be able to be identified. Other patient factors include poor tissue healing due to deficient or defective collagen, smoking, mesh shrinkage, steroid usage, aging, etc. The operations to repair a recurrence will be selected by the surgeon. Generally, if the laparoscopic repair was performed, many surgeons would elect to operate via the open method. This will allow the surgery to occur in non-scarred tissues away from the iliac vessels where the mesh was placed during the initial procedure. However, the use of the MIS approach is not always absolutely contraindicated in such a situation.

## Ventral and Incisional Hernia Surgery

The MIS approach to these hernias is grown slowly over the years since the first procedure was performed. This is in large part to the limitations of the laparoscopic instrumentation initially. Subsequently, this "new" technique required a learning curve that older surgeons were not willing to undertake. Currently, this procedure is taught to residents and is used following their training. There are fellowships in MIS surgery as well. As discussed previously, if a patient can tolerate a general anesthetic, this can be an option. There is a particular outcome benefit to this approach in the obese patient [16]. Recent data confirms that there is a shorter operative time, lower length of hospital stay, and overall lower institutional costs associated with laparoscopic repair compared to the open repair of incisional hernias [17].

Preoperatively if there is question of the location and size of the hernia(s), a CT scan is appropriate. It is sometimes impossible to identify the borders of the hernia in an obese patient. The location of the hernia will significantly influence the location of trocars to perform the operation. This CT scan, unfortunately, will not aid in the identification of any adhesions that may be present within the abdomen. It can identify the contents of the hernia effectively. It is most helpful to use both oral (especially) and intravenous contrast to do this examination. Additionally, this scan should include both the abdomen and pelvis, as this is necessary to evaluate the entire contents of the abdomen. Not uncommonly, a hernia that was unsuspected will also be identified. This could be repaired concomitantly to the presenting fascial defect. Other preoperative considerations were discussed earlier in this chapter.

Large fascial defects that have more of the abdominal contents in the hernia than inside the abdomen are not candidates for this method. Areas of very thin skin with or without skin breakdown or a prior split thickness skin graft directly over intestine should not be selected either. These areas of skin are likely to necrose if the bowel is removed from the skin because it may draw blood supply from the intestine. Ascites is a relative contraindication, but portal venous hypertension is considered a contraindication. Interestingly, a small individual with a moderate- to large-sized defect may not be a good candidate due to the required size of mesh needed to properly repair the hernia. This will make the procedure difficult due to the lateral placement might imped the use of the lateral trocar locations.

While the typical uncomplicated laparoscopic inguinal hernia may take 45–90 min, these procedures can take 3–4 h to complete. This will be influenced by the severity of any adhesions that are present from prior operations, the presence and location of any prior mesh material, and the size of the patient. Nearly all of these patients will require both a nasogastric tube and urinary drainage catheter unless the hernia to be repaired is relatively small. Central venous and/or arterial monitoring lines are generally not necessary in the operating room.

Patient positioning in the surgical suite will vary according to the location of the hernia, the size of the patient, and whether or not a robot will be used. The arms are preferably tucked to allow access to the entire abdominal surface, but this cannot be done in large individuals. The use of Trendelenburg or reverse Trendelenburg positions will frequently be required as well. The surgeons and assistants will stand on either side of the patient for the laparoscopic method. For lateral hernias such as a flank hernia, the patient may have to be placed on a roll to maintain a slight or full lateral decubitus position.

There is a large variation of trocar sizes and positions that will be used by the surgeon. The items discussed above, too, will influence these options. In general,

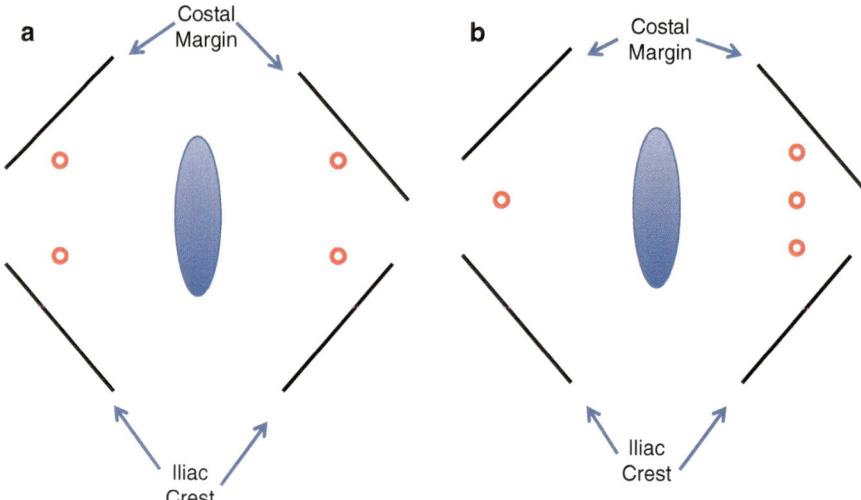

**Fig. 12.13** (**a**, **b**) Trocar positions for laparoscopic incisional hernia repair. The blue oval represents the midline hernia. The red circles represent trocar sites

four trocars will be used. These can be positioned with two on both sides of the abdomen or three on one side with another on the opposite location (Fig. 12.13a, b). Four trocars will suffice in most patients; however, the surgeon may find it advantageous to place additional trocars to facilitate the performance of a safe and effective operation. The robotic approach will access the patient from only one side where all trocars are placed on the side opposite the robot itself.

The most risky and challenging portion of these procedures is the actual adhesiolysis to expose the hernia(s). There are many different methods with this to carry out this portion of the procedure. Of greatest concern is the potential of an injury to the intestine, which has a mortality rate of 6–9% in a series of patients but it is as high as 40% if unrecognized [18, 19]. Surgical options to lyse these adhesions include the use of electrocautery, ultrasonic dissection, or bipolar dissection. Many surgeons elect to use no energy source at all to lessen the risk of intestinal injury. If there is a significant amount of adhesiolysis, the patient can experience a prolonged ileus that frequently requires a nasogastric tube for a few days postoperatively to decompress the stomach.

Once the lysis of adhesions has been accomplished, the fascial defect(s) will be measured. This measurement will dictate the size of the mesh selected. The distance covered past the edges of the defect determines the size of mesh needed. This is called mesh overlap. In most cases, the preferred overlap of the fascial defect will be 5 cm or more. This has been shown to lower the rate of recurrence [20]. In other words, if the defect is 5 cm × 5 cm, the selected mesh will be 15 cm × 15 cm to provide 5 cm overlap in all directions. Other considerations have recently been described to aid in the sizing of mesh overlap [21, 22].

A relatively recent development has been the closure of the fascial defect prior to mesh placement. The increased use of the surgical robot has brought this to the forefront, as it is much easier to accomplish this using this technology. This can also be accomplished with the traditional MIS methods albeit with more difficulty. The perceived benefit to closure is the potential to decrease recurrence rates and seroma rates and improve ingrowth into the mesh material [23]. If this is selected, the patients can experience more pain in the midline (or where the hernia exists) than if it is not closed. This is still a controversial subject.

The prosthetic material will be placed and fixed to the anterior abdominal wall by a variety of methods. One of the many fixation devices can be used (described earlier in the chapter) with or without the use of transfascial sutures. Transfascial sutures are actually placed trans-abdominally rather than through the inner layer of fascia. They are placed via a skin incision through all of the layers of the abdominal wall using a "suture passing" instrument. Various numbers of them will be used from a minimum of four to ten or more depending on the decision of the surgeon, the size of the hernia, and/or mesh. These can result in pain at these sites for months or longer. Occasionally they must be removed due to chronic pain. In the typical robot-assisted surgery, the mesh is sewn directly onto the fascia of the innermost layer, the transversus abdominis fascia, and muscle. These patients may experience more pain initially, but it usually does not persist as long as with the transfascial suture.

The length of stay in the hospital will vary depending on the comorbidities of the patient, the difficulty with adhesiolysis, postoperative pain, and the perceived risk of enterotomy. Intuitively, the smaller hernias will allow for an earlier discharge than the large hernias with incarcerated contents and significant adhesions. An early indicator of an intestinal injury is an increased amount of abdominal pain, significant free intra-abdominal air, an increased white blood cell count or band count, and tachycardia. If these conditions exist, a need for further workup is indicated, or the patient can be returned to the operating room for a diagnostic laparoscopy.

Recovery from this procedure differs significantly from patient to patient. Many factors will impact the length of time needed, many of which are not related to the operation itself and beyond the control of the physicians. The exact method of repair will impact this to some extent. Most patients will be allowed to increase their activity level as the pain allows. Although there is still need of more data, it appears the robotically assisted repair allows for a slightly shorter recovery.

A very common occurrence is the development of a postoperative seroma at the site of the hernia itself. This is more likely if the peritoneal sac of the hernia is not removed. It generally is never removed due to the risk of postoperative hemorrhage at the site. If the fascial defect is not closed, this is also more frequently seen. In most instances, simple observation will suffice, as the majority will resolve in a few weeks or months. The use of an abdominal binder postoperatively seems to aid in the resolution of the fluid collection. Infrequently these are a cosmetic issue that does not resolve, and interventional radiology can place a drain into the seroma to treat it. One must accept the risk of an infection if this is undertaken. Rarely, if this persists, the patient must be taken to the operating room for surgical excision of the seroma and the persistent capsule that surrounds it.

The issues noted for inguinal hernias increase the risk of recurrence, but these factors are an even greater consideration in the incisional and ventral hernias. The rate of recurrence for the laparoscopic repair varies from 0% to 11% in most series. The more experience that the surgeon possesses, the lower the rate. In the event of a suspected recurrence, a CT scan should be done. It should be noted that most mesh materials are not visible on a CT scan [24]. If a recurrence is verified, the patient can undergo another attempt of the MIS repair, or the open repair may be the better approach. There are many options for the open repair such as a traditional repair or one that involves the "component separation" in which the fascial layers are divided to allow for re-approximation of the midline. These methods are beyond the scope of this chapter.

## Robotic Hernia Surgery

The surgical robot has been available for many years and is especially well known in the gynecologic and urologic specialties. A common misconception is that the robot is a true new method of surgery. In fact, the robot is merely a different method of the control of the laparoscopic instrumentation used by the surgeon. As noted earlier, the surgeon stands at the bedside of the operating table during laparoscopic surgery. The robot is controlled by the surgeon who sits at a console at some distance from the operating table. In both options, the ultimate control of the operation remains with the surgeon. There is no computer that operates the robot other than that which allows the surgeon to control the computer that supports the robot.

The Intuitive Surgical (Sunnyvale, CA, USA) robot was approved for hernia repair in 2014. This has allowed the robotic surgeons to repair hernias with the benefits of the degrees of freedom of the instrumentation that is not available with traditional laparoscopic instruments. Additionally, the optics with the robot is three rather than two-dimensional. Data is still needed, but it appears that this represents an improvement in surgical technique [25]. It is anticipated that in the next year or two, other surgical robots will be available to the surgeon. While each may provide differing operative advantages, the overall concept to repair hernias will likely be unaffected.

Cost increases due to the robot are often cited as a reason to not implement its use for any operation. It is true that disregard of the utilization of instruments will increase costs. Most surgeons, however, are quite aware that frugal use of them will help prevent cost concerns. Aside from the capital outlay, the business decision to purchase a surgical robot should be reflective of the benefits that result from its use. There is still a huge amount of discussion amongst surgeons on this topic. I truly believe that the costs can be lower than traditional open surgery due to the decrease in the length of stay in the hospital. The long-term outcomes that we are currently witnessing justify its use. More data will confirm this in the future.

## Miscellaneous Considerations

There are a few other concerns that should be mentioned in the context of this chapter. For instance, the selection of the mesh material may not be at the sole discretion of the surgeon. Currently, many hospital systems use large purchasing groups to buy supplies at reduced costs. This often impacts the availability of the products that surgeons are allowed access in the operating room. This will greatly impact the types and brands of laparoscopic equipment and most importantly the types and sizes of mesh materials that can be selected. Depending on the location within any country, the mesh available may or may not be the one that the surgeon desires. This can affect outcomes to some degree.

In any operating room, the necessary personnel will influence the flow and pace of all operations. This is especially important in the MIS arena and is even more acute with the surgical robot. The use of the advanced instrumentation requires trouble shooting by the nurses related to the computers, insufflators, electrocautery, and other devices that are required by the surgeon. Highly skilled personnel are critical to the success of these procedures. Additionally, the knowledge of the variety of mesh products and even the location of them within the confines of the surgical suites necessitates highly skilled nurses. These people are often overlooked in the MIS area, but they remain critical components of the operations.

## Conclusion

Minimally invasive surgery in the field of hernia repair is gaining in its influence in the general surgery field. The robotic repair has greatly increased the adoption of this technology for these operations. It is not infrequent that patients are requesting these methods. The internist should maintain a general knowledge of the MIS approach to hernia repair to understand and advice patients. This chapter represents an introduction to this option in the repair of hernias.

## References

1. Kirkpatrick T, Allain BW, LeBlanc KA. Laparoscopic inguinal hernia repair. In: KA LB, Kingsnorth AN, Sanders D, editors. Management of abdominal wall hernias. 5th ed: Springer; In press.
2. LeBlanc KA, Booth WV. Laparoscopic repair of incisional abdominal hernias using expanded polytetrafluoroethylene: preliminary findings. Surg Lap Endo. 1993;3(1):39–41.
3. Liang MK, Holihan JL, Itani K, et al. Ventral hernia management: expert consensus guided by systematic review. Ann Surg. 2017;265(1):80–9.
4. Luijendijk RW, Hop WC, van den Tol MP, et al. A comparison of suture repair with mesh repair for incisional hernia. N Engl J Med. 2000;343(6):392–8.
5. Burger JW, Luijendijk RW. Hop et al. long-term follow-up of a randomized controlled trial of suture versus mesh repair of incisional hernia. Ann Surg. 2004;240(4):578–83; discussion 583–5.
6. LeBlanc KA. Prostheses and products for hernioplasty. In: KA LB, Kingsnorth AN, Sanders D, editors. Management of abdominal wall hernias. 5th ed: Springer; In press.
7. Rosen MJ, Bauer JJ, Harmaty M, Carbonell AM, Cobb WS, Matthews B, Goldblatt MI, Selzer DJ, Poulose BK, Hansson BME, Rosman C, Chao JJ, Jacobsen GR. Multicenter, prospective

longitudinal study of the recurrence, surgical site infection, and quality of life after contaminated ventral hernia repair using biosynthetic absorbable mesh. Ann Surg. 2017;265:205–11.

8. McCormack K, Scott N, Go PM, Ross SJ, Grant A, Collaboration of EU Hernia Trialists. Laparoscopic techniques versus open techniques for inguinal hernia repair. Cochrane Database Syst Rev. 2003;1: Art. No:CD001785. https://doi.org/10.1002/14651858.

9. Roll S, Skinovsky J. Laparoscopic TAPP inguinal hernia repair. In: Novitsky YW, editor. Hernia surgery – current principles. Cham: Springer; 2016. p. 451–60.

10. Kindel T, Oleynikov D. Laparoscopic total extra-peritoneal (TEP) inguinal hernia repair. In: Novitsky YW, editor. Hernia surgery – current principles. Cham: Springer; 2016. p. 461–6.

11. Topart P, Vandenbroucke F, Lozac'h P. Tisseel versus tack staples as mesh fixation in totally extraperitoneal laparoscopic repair of groin hernias: a retrospective analysis. Surg Endosc. 2005;19(5):724 7.

12. Taylor C, Layani L, Liew V, Ghusn M, Crampton N, White S. Laparoscopic inguinal hernia repair without mesh fixation, early results of a large randomized clinical trial. Surg Endosc. 2008;22(3):757–62.

13. Hallén M, Sevonius D, Westerdahl J, Gunnarsson U, Sandblom G. Risk factors for reoperation due to chronic groin postherniorrhaphy pain. Hernia. 2015;19:863–9.

14. Belyansky I, Tsirline VB, Klima DA, Walters AL, Lincourt AE, Heniford T. Prospective, comparative study of postoperative quality of life in TEP, TAPP, and modified Lichtenstein repairs. Ann Surg. 2011;254:709–15.

15. Carter NH, Chen DC. Chronic pain after inguinal repair. In: KA LB, Kingsnorth AN, Sanders D, editors. Management of abdominal wall hernias. 5th ed: Springer; In press.

16. Novitsky YW, Cobb WS, Kercher KW, Matthews BD, Sing RF, Heniford BT. Laparoscopic ventral hernia repair in obese patients: a new standard of care. Arch Surg. 2006;141(1):57–61.

17. Soliani G, De Troia A, Protinari M, Targa S, Carcoforo P, Vasquez G, Fisichella PM, Feo CV. Laparoscopic versus open incisional hernia repair: a retrospective cohort study with costs analysis on 269 patients. Hernia. 2017;21:609–18.

18. Elieson MJ, Corder JM, LeBlanc KA. Enterotomy and mortality rates of laparoscopic incisional and ventral hernia repair: a review of the literature. JSLS. 2007;11:408–14.

19. Sharma A, Khullar R, Soni V, Baijal M, Kapahi A, Najma K, Chowbey PK. Iatrogenic enterotomy in laparoscopic ventral/incisional hernia repair: a single center experience of 2,346 patients over 17 years. Hernia. 2013;17(5):581–7.

20. LeBlanc KA. Mesh overlap is a key determinant of hernia recurrence following laparoscopic ventral and incisional hernia repair. Hernia. 2016;20(1):85–9.

21. Tulloh B, de Beaux A. Defects and donuts: the importance of the mesh:defect area ratio. Hernia. 2016;20:893–5.

22. Hauters P, Desmet J, Gherardi D, Dewaele S, Poilvache H, Malvaux P. Assessment of predictive factors for recurrence in laparoscopic ventral hernia repair using a bridging technique. Surg Endosc. 2017;31:3656. https://doi.org/10.1007/s00464-016-5401-0.

23. Tandon A, Pathak S, Lyons NJ, Nunes QM, Daniels IR, Smart NJ. Meta-analysis of closure of the fascial defect during laparoscopic incisional and ventral hernia repair. Br J Surg. 2016;103(12):1598–607.

24. Rakic S, LeBlanc KA. The radiologic appearance of prosthetic materials use in hernia repair and a recommended classification. AJR. 2013;201(6):11890–3.

25. Gonzales A, Escobar E, Romero R, Walker G, Mejias J, Gallas M, Dickens E, Johnson CJ, Rabaza J, Kudsi OY. Robotic-assisted ventral hernia repair: a multicenter evaluation of clinical outcomes. Surg Endosc. 2017;31(3):1342–9.

# Index

© Springer Nature Switzerland AG 2019
C. Rezac, K. Donohue (eds.), *The Internist's Guide to Minimally Invasive
Gastrointestinal Surgery*, Clinical Gastroenterology,
https://doi.org/10.1007/978-3-319-96631-1

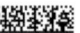